Antibodies and Immunity

Books by G. J. V. Nossal

Antigens, Lymphoid Cells and the Immune Response
(with G. L. Ada)

Medical Science and Human Goals

ANTIBODIES AND IMMUNITY

G. J. V. NOSSAL

SECOND, REVISED

AND EXPANDED EDITION

BASIC BOOKS, INC., PUBLISHERS

NEW YORK

For Katrina, Michael, Brigid, and Stephen

Library of Congress Cataloging in Publication Data

Nossal, Gustav Joseph Victor, 1931–
  Antibodies and immunity.

  Includes index.
  1. Immunology.   I.   Title.
QR181.N67   1978   616.07'9   77-75251
ISBN 0-465-00361-3

Contents

List of Figures

Preface to the Second Edition

WHEN I first wrote *Antibodies and Immunity* in 1968, my primary aim was to capture the fascination and promise of the subject of immunology in a form intelligible to the non-scientist, with virtually no background knowledge of biology. To my surprise and delight, the first edition won the Phi Beta Kappa Science Award, indicating that I may, to a degree, have succeeded in my purpose. A second surprise dawned more slowly, and this was the progressive realization that the book, in its original English version and in its German, Italian, and Russian translations, was being extensively used by students of biology and medicine. While in no sense a textbook, it has apparently served to introduce the subject to undergraduates in a readily digestible, yet responsible way, making later formal study less of a chore. It was the increasingly frequent pleadings by my academic colleagues for an updating that has provided the main motivation for a second edition.

In the nine years that have passed, a very great deal of new knowledge has accumulated in immunology, and its "second golden age" shows no signs of falling into decline. This has posed something of a dilemma. Obviously, the new knowledge has to be included, but I felt it important to preserve the readability of the book, achieved chiefly by the use of rather homely analogies, and also its brevity. These conflicting aims could not be achieved through anything short of a total rewriting. In this second version, I have again risked the ire of my colleagues by omitting the qualifications and exceptions which are so essential in a formal scientific treatise. In fact, I derive some satisfaction from having exceeded the first edition's length only slightly, despite having included material from some very recent international conferences.

Of the many new perspectives which have emerged in the last decade, four warrant special mention: discovery of the nature and functions of the cell membrane; realization of the elaborate interactions occurring between T and B lymphocytes; genetics of the major histocompatibility locus and of immune responses; and the new excitement about tropical parasitic diseases. These areas have been covered in Chapters 13, 9, 15, and 21, respectively. The interplay between cells once thought to be quite independent of one another has also necessitated a great deal of reordering of material; the information on the thymus, thymus-derived cells and cell-mediated immunity are now placed much earlier in the book. Reluctantly, some older data have had to be considerably compressed. The material of the former Chapter 14 on "The Wandering Lymphocyte" has been incorporated into the present Chapters 4 and 7, and that of the former Chapter 21 on "Irradiation" into Chapters 10 and 20.

Two other changes should improve the value of the book for students. The illustrations have been redrawn to give better quality and detail; and a guide to further reading has been included. I also wish to record my thanks to the many colleagues who have sent comments about the first edition, offering criticisms or pointing out errors missed in proofreading. Usually (not always!) they were right and their help has improved the volume.

My sincere thanks are due to Miss N. O'Neill for her patient and efficient typing of the manuscript, to Dr. J. Goding, Dr. G. Gutman, Dr. T. Mandel, Dr. J. F. A. P. Miller and Dr. M. Schumacher for contributing new figures and redesigning others for this edition, to Miss C. Gichard for editorial assistance, and to Mr. R. Mahony and Miss S. Belan for help in reproducing the figures. Original studies reported in Chapters 2, 4, and 5–13 were supported by grants and contracts from the National Health and Medical Research Council, Canberra, Australia; the National Institutes of Health grant AI-O-3958; and were in part pursuant to contract number NIH–NCI–7–3889 with the National Cancer Institute. This is publication number 2304 from the Walter and Eliza Hall Institute of Medical Research.

G. J. V. Nossal
Melbourne, January 1977

Antibodies and Immunity

1

FASCINATIONS AND FRUITS
OF TWO GOLDEN AGES

THE CEASELESS, cruel, yet richly productive process of evolution has given us the phenomenon of man. With thoughtless arrogance we assume ourselves to represent the pinnacle in biological achievement. Yet, despite the extraordinary control over environmental forces which our species gained over the millennia, one specter, with incalculable effects on the course of history, remained a daily threat to human happiness and survival right up to the present century. This was infectious disease, and especially epidemic disease. The bacteria and viruses responsible for plague, typhoid, cholera, smallpox, and poliomyelitis represented enemies more subtle and more dangerous than the elements or the larger predators. To the historians of the future, the virtual elimination of the major infectious diseases as significant causes of death in Western communities will surely rank as one of the key signposts of this extraordinary century. This conquest can be ascribed to the parallel development of the twin sciences microbiology and immunology.

The first "golden age of immunology," in fact, had its roots in the latter part of the nineteenth century. This was the era of Louis Pasteur and rabies vaccination, von Behring and Wernicke with their anti-diphtheria sera, and Ehrlich and Metchnikoff probing the theoretical aspects of bodily defenses. The first two decades of the twentieth century saw a rapid practical expansion of immunization procedures and remarkable progress in experimentation on antibodies, the protective protein molecules poured into the bloodstream after vaccination. By the mid–1930s, immunization had gained wide public acceptance and the spotlight in disease control shifted to the sulphonamides and soon to the even more magical antibiotics. A medical student introduced to bacteriology in 1950, as I was, might have been excused for thinking that the heyday of immunology was over. In fact, quite the reverse was true, as this decade marked the beginning of the second golden age of immunology, which is currently still in a phase of ascendancy.

To what can we ascribe this rebirth of interest in immune mechanisms? The reasons are both medical and scientific. From the medical viewpoint, it has become clear that the cells and molecules of the immune system are by no means solely concerned with infectious or epidemic diseases, important though these are. For example, the immune system attempts to defend the body against cancer and the spread of malignant cells around the body. It can foil the endeavors of the surgeon who transplants organs to replace diseased ones. The same types of cells that react aggressively to foreign microbes recognize the foreignness of the organ graft. Unless stopped by treatments which will be described, these lymphocyte cells will rapidly kill the transplant. This uncanny capacity of the lymphocytes to discriminate between "self" and "not self" is still the subject of intensive research. Immune cells are prominently involved in inflammation and tissue repair. A large part of the field of clinical immunology is concerned with what happens when the immune system goes wrong in some way. This can happen when some infectious agent is too clever for the immune system and persists despite the latter's best efforts. The antibodies attach to molecules made by the invader, and the resulting immune complexes can have serious irritating effects on many tissues, particularly if they remain present for long periods. In other cases, inherent faults appear in the immune system, and "bad" antibodies are made. These include antibodies to normally harmless substances like grasses or pollens which cause allergies, or antibodies to vital constituents of the body itself, which cause serious or even fatal diseases termed autoimmune diseases. Obviously, better understanding of the functioning of the immune system will have great impact on the whole fabric of medicine. Increasing the destruction of cancer cells by stimulating the patient's immune system; decreasing the invasion of grafts to allow successful "spare parts" surgery; controlling immune processes in autoimmunity and allergy; these are some of the daily, and hopefully not too distant, pipe dreams of the modern immunologist, and we shall look at the efforts to make them come true.

The more academic reasons for the immunology research explosion are no less compelling. The central fascination concerns the immune system as a *molecular learning system.* Antibody molecules of bewilderingly diverse shapes are made individually and differently by each animal, reflecting its history of exposure to the microbial world and the environment. This process at first sight appears to be so different from the conventional norm where proteins, the key molecular machines of living matter, are made to a rigid pattern dictated by the structure of the DNA blueprints, the gene for that protein. We now know a good deal about information flow from the DNA template, via the intermediate molecule called messenger RNA, to the final protein product. The shape of a protein and its properties is determined by the number and sequential arrangement of 20 kinds of building blocks, the amino acids. How can the body, with a limited number of genes for antibody proteins, produce an apparently infinite variety of antibody molecules patterned to fit exactly to the particular antigen (or vaccine substance) eliciting the particular immune response? This apparent exception to the central dogma of molecular biology and evolution (that information flows from DNA to RNA to protein and not in the reverse direction) represents the kind of brainteaser that scientists love as a challenge. While far from the final answer, we have made good progress towards understanding this and have revealed unique mechanisms of great interest.

Another area of marked progress has been in the regulation of the immune response. When antigens enter the body, they stimulate lymphocytes and make them divide repeatedly. How does the body ensure that this process starts efficiently, and stops in time before the teeming billions of lymphocytes overgrow the other blood cells and cause leukemia? How does the healthy immune system stop itself from reacting to bodily antigens? All of this depends on subtle interplay between the individual cells, which, like people in a civilized society, do not lead entirely independent lives but rather influence one another and display multiple mutual dependencies. These regulations and interactions occupy center stage in immunology research today.

A further explanation of the immunology boom is more general: it concerns the importance of model-building in science. The central desire of every biologist is to gain deeper insight into the life process. As each scientist recognizes the impossibility of integrating all the known biological facts into one human mind, he or she strives to build models. This involves taking a particular phenomenon (be it the division of a bacterium, the beat of an isolated frog's heart, or the effect of a light beam on a cat's retina) and studying it in minute detail, not only because of its intrinsic interest, but because it may bring out some general biological principle. The wonderful progress that has been made in biology in the last quarter century has depended on such model-building. The validity of attempts at integration has been underscored by the recognition of the essential unity of all living matter. The same genetic code, the same basic principles of energy generation, the same overall rules of cellular organization are shared throughout the plant and animal kingdoms. For a variety of historical and operational reasons, the immune system of mammals has been chosen by many researchers as a model system for probing into the mysteries of living cells in general.

There are hopes that understanding the basis of immune memory and learning may stimulate concepts in the still more complex learning processes of the brain. Cell-cell interaction in immunology is watched closely by students of differentiation—the way by which a few cells in the early embryo move away from one another and construct the separate parts of the body. The reproduction of lymphocytes represents a kind of Darwinian evolution in a microcosm and is thereby relevant to advances in genetics. In these respects, immunology is a unifying force in biology today, attracting devotees from many specialties.

One frequently hears the criticism about research workers that they are simply learning more and more about less and less, and the fear about science in general that it will disintegrate into a vast collection of introverted, unconnected subspecialties. The triumphs of molecular and cell biology, genetics, and immunology over recent years have shown that nothing could be further from the truth.

In this book we will look first at what is known about antibodies and the cells that make them. Only when we have a reasonable knowledge of the normal functioning of the immune system will we turn our attention to the practical implications of this knowledge for human medicine. I hope every reader will draw from this sequence a conclusion which should be self-evident but is all too frequently forgotten. There can be no rational diagnosis, no improvement in human health, without the presence of a substantial foundation of detailed knowledge of how things work before they go wrong. As a full-time medical researcher, who sees few patients, I am frequently asked to explain exactly what I do. The casual questioner, when told I am in research, will then usually ask, "Oh, you're looking for a cure for cancer—or is it the common cold?" Nearly always he is reluctant to accept the possibility that someone who is trained as a doctor can spend his days and nights worrying about how cells from perfectly healthy mice make antibodies. He is surprised, not to say dismayed, that well over 50 percent of current medical research is of a similar nature. "Wasn't the body's normal functioning all wrapped up years ago?" he will ask. In fact, our knowledge of the normal is increasing daily, and only on this knowledge can we build the medical miracles of the future.

2

ANTIGENS

AN eighteenth-century English milkmaid unwittingly discovered the first useful *antigen*. She pointed out to the English general practitioner, Edward Jenner, the odd observation that milkmaids who had caught cowpox (vaccinia) from a member of her herd never subsequently came down with the dreaded smallpox (variola). Jenner was impressed, and intrepidly tested her theory. He inoculated human beings with fluid from a cowpox sore, which resulted in a mild condition only. Indeed, the treatment conferred protection from the infinitely more serious related disorder. Although these studies were well documented and controlled, they were a real shot in the dark. Jenner lived in an age when no one knew about viruses or the true nature of infections. For this reason immunity research lay static for a century, in fact until our first golden age. However, so important historically and practically was Jenner's work that we have come loosely to term all immunization procedures by the word which describes Jenner's procedure—vaccination. The first vaccine contained vaccinia virus—though Jenner didn't know it. Present-day vaccines contain a large variety of different molecules which call forth production of complementary anti-

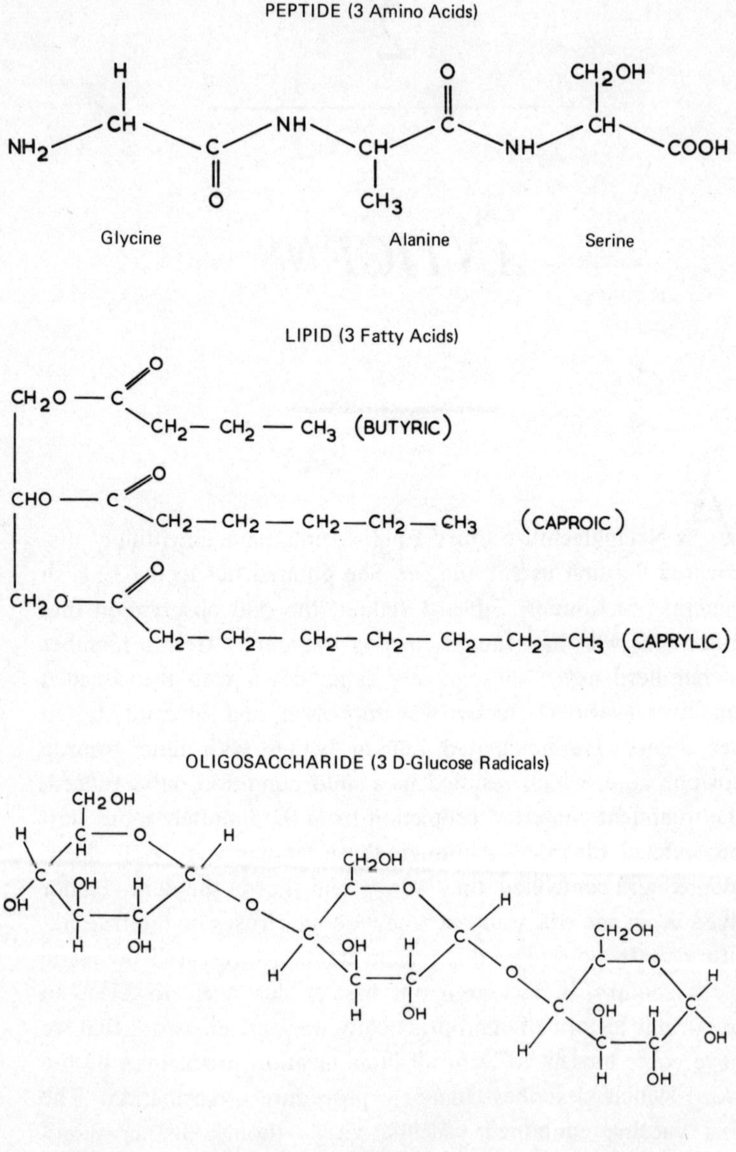

Figure 2–1. Chemical composition of some important cell building blocks.

bodies. Because they *generate* antibody production, we call these molecules *antigens*. This chapter will deal with the nature of antigens and will, perhaps, explain why Jenner's experiment worked.

It is perhaps fitting that the revision of this chapter is taking place during the very weeks in 1976 that a World Health Organization team, under Dr. D. A. Henderson, is eliminating the last few reservoirs of the smallpox virus from remote Ethiopian villages. This total eradication of smallpox from the world is proof that the inheritors of the Jennerian legacy have not been idle!

What Is an Antigen?

Living cells are made up of many different compounds, including water, minerals, small organic molecules such as hormones and vitamins, and a host of other materials. However, the most characteristic molecules of living forms are the four great families of *macromolecules*: proteins, carbohydrates, lipids, and nucleic acids. These are big molecules, composed of many smaller parts; in other words, they are *polymers*. The chemical formulas of some of the building blocks of these organic polymers are shown in Figure 2–1. Proteins are made up of amino acids, carbohydrates of sugars, and lipids or fats of glycerol and fatty acids. Nucleic acids are more complex and consist of units called *nucleotides* strung together; each nucleotide consists of a phosphate group, a sugar, and a base. Their structure and function will be considered again in Chapter 4.

We can symbolically show the formulas of these molecules by drawing them on a piece of paper. However, we must remember that in reality they are three-dimensional, and are better visualized as in Figure 2–2. If we think, in three-dimensional terms, of a portion of a macromolecule consisting of three to ten

METHANE MOLECULE

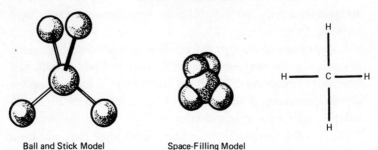

Ball and Stick Model   Space-Filling Model

Figure 2–2. Building block in three-dimensional terms. The ball-and-stick model shows clearly the angles between the different bonds of the molecule. However, the bonded atoms are not really spherical in shape, nor are they separated in space by rigid bonds. The space-filling model (called the Van der Waals model) shows to scale the relative size of each atom, but the bond angles and bond distances are more difficult to see. One uses whichever model is more appropriate for one's purpose.

average-sized building blocks such as sugars or amino acids, we obtain a picture of one unit of antigen, or in technical terms, one *antigenic determinant*. It is an area or contour of this size which locks with one molecule of antibody, as we shall see in Chapter 3. Virtually no work of an immunological nature has been done with fats, but each of the other three classes of macromolecules can act as antigens. Now as one molecule of protein, for example, can contain hundreds or even thousands of component amino-acid units, clearly a single molecule of antigen can, and usually does, contain a number of antigenic determinants. We are now in a position to define our terms: An *antigenic determinant* is a molecule or portion of a molecule capable of binding firmly to the combining site of an antibody; an *antigen* is a molecule containing one or more antigenic determinants.

Though most of the antigens in nature are proteins or carbohydrates, it would be misleading to suggest that no other chemical configurations are antigenic. In fact, chemists can hook quite small molecules, termed *haptens*, to a protein "carrier." When this hapten-protein conjugate is injected into an animal, a variety of antibodies are formed. Some of these recognize and unite with the "carrier" portion, others with the hapten. Almost any type of chemical can act as a hapten, or in other words it is possible to make antibodies against almost anything. The exception is that animals cannot make antibodies against certain of their own bodily constituents, and we will have occasion to return to this point a number of times.

The Concept of Immunogenicity

So far we have described antigens simply in terms of their test-tube behavior—their ability to lock to antibody molecules. Another property of antigens, not possessed by all, is the capacity to call forth antibody production. This property we describe with the clumsy word "immunogenicity." Let us take a simple example. One protein known to most people is egg white, technically known as ovalbumin. Like most proteins, ovalbumin is an antigen; that is, it can react with specific antibody molecules directed against it. The serum of a normal rabbit will not contain antibodies to ovalbumin. When we inject a solution of ovalbumin under the skin of the rabbit, it will, within a few days, make specific antibody, and if we bleed it the serum will contain numerous molecules of antiovalbumin. Therefore, the ovalbumin is *immunogenic* in the rabbit. However, if we inject ovalbumin into a normal chicken, we are injecting one of the chicken's own bodily constituents, and no antibody formation results. In other words, the ovalbumin is not immunogenic in the chicken. Similarly, small molecules can be antigenic, but, with some exceptions, molecules smaller than molecular weight 3,000 are not immunogenic unless they are hooked onto a larger carrier molecule. The distinction may seem academic, but unless these two separate properties of antigen molecules are made clear, confusion could arise in our later discussions.

Synthetic Antigens

Most immunologists work with antigens derived from some natural source such as animal tissues or microbes. However, organic chemists have learned to synthesize protein and carbohydrate antigens in the test tube, starting with simple sugars or amino acids as building blocks. Studies with these artificial antigens have taught us much about the nature of both antigenicity and immunogenicity. For example, they have shown us the size of an antigenic determinant and have demonstrated that certain sugars and amino acids contribute more to a molecule's immunogenicity than others. This is mentioned here because we are about to embark on a discussion of useful vaccines. Surprisingly, very few modern immunologists (in this second golden age) use these vaccines in their research. They are more likely to choose some esoteric, highly pure material, the composition of which is much more accurately defined than even the purest commercial vaccine. Each vaccine consists of multiple proteins, and most proteins of a mosaic of antigenic determinants. Synthetic antigens can be made with little or no heterogeneity of antigenic determinants, a property the full value of which we will recognize in Chapter 15.

Vaccines

We have seen that a single antigenic determinant is only a small portion of an antigen molecule. Similarly, a single antigen molecule is only a minute fraction of a pathogenic microbe. A small virus particle, such as poliomyelitis, contains many different kinds of antigens, and thousands of molecules of each kind. A single bacterium, such as a typhoid bacillus, contains many more. A preparation containing antigens from microbes or microbial products, useful in the prevention of some infectious diseases, is known as a vaccine.

Vaccines fall into three general classes. The simplest to understand is the class exemplified by Salk vaccine. This consists of poliomyelitis virus particles that have been killed by formalin. Obviously, a dead virus cannot multiply and infect a living host. However, provided care is taken in the killing process, the antigen molecules of a virus or bacterium are not significantly affected. When injected into a person, they are immunogenic and cause antibody production even though no infection results from their injection. The commonest vaccines in this class are those against typhoid, paratyphoid A and B, cholera, whooping cough, and some forms of polio vaccine.

In the second class of vaccines the antigen consists not of the whole microbe but of modified poisonous material made by that microbe. For example, diphtheria bacilli multiply predominantly in the throat. Here they do some damage locally, which is reflected in the exudate seen at the back of the throat. This is of little importance compared with their capacity to secrete, while they grow, a poison known as diphtheria toxin. This travels in the bloodstream and has many bad effects on the body, including a paralyzing action on the heart muscles. Quite small doses can kill a child. Again, fairly mild chemical treatments can detoxify such poisons. For example, gentle heat and formalin treatment can change diphtheria toxin into a harmless "toxoid," which has lost its pharmacological power but retains its immunogenicity. Apart from diphtheria toxoid, the most commonly used vaccine of this sort is tetanus toxoid.

The third type of vaccine is perhaps the best of all. It is termed a *live, attenuated* vaccine. Such vaccines consist of living bacteria or viruses which actually infect and multiply in the tissues of the host. However, they are really only cousins of the natural, virulent microbes. By laboratory manipulations, generally involving growth of the microbe in a strange environment, the immunologist has produced genetic variants of the original strain. These are antigenically similar to the disease-causing organism, but lack much or all of their ancestor's virulence. Examples of this class are Sabin-type oral polio vaccine, BCG vaccine against tuberculosis, and injectable antiviral vaccines such as measles, German measles, or smallpox. The advantage of these agents over the other two types is that they simulate a natural infection. Some multiplication of the organism in the body takes place, and this magnifies the antigenic stimulus. Frequently, one vaccination with a living agent can achieve as much antibody production as three or four injections of a killed vaccine. In the case of the Sabin vaccine, even the needle prick is saved. The living virus is given by mouth and multiplies inside the gut. However, it has lost completely the power to penetrate into nervous tissue, and thus cannot cause paralysis.

We now return to our fabled milkmaid. Inadvertently, she had noted an *antigenic relationship* between the vaccinia and variola viruses. Though by no means identical, these two viruses share certain antigenic determinants. They are sufficiently similar in that antibodies made against one will prevent the multiplication of the other. Although the crude cowpox fluid used by Jenner was less refined than the present vaccine lymph, the basic principle of this form of immunization remains unchanged.

The Future of Vaccination

In Chapter 1 we hinted that some of the gloss had vanished from the field of vaccination, at least from the theoretician's viewpoint. While it is true that other branches of immunology are currently more fashionable, it should be remembered that immunization still abounds with challenges for the future. For example, no vaccines exist for the great parasitic scourges of tropical climates, such as malaria, schistosomiasis or snail fever, African sleeping sickness, or elephantiasis and river blindness caused by filarial worms (this important field is covered in Chapter 21). In developed countries, some common infections remain to plague us, including the common cold, infectious hepatitis (jaundice), and venereal diseases. Some of the vaccines that we do have are not nearly as effective as they ought to be, and intensive research on better, longer lasting cholera, typhoid, and influenza vaccines is proceeding. Most vaccines have side effects, usually mild (such as a sore gland in the armpit or a slight fever) but occasionally severe. At least a proportion of these ought to be preventable by purer vaccines. New techniques of genetic engineering have even raised the hope that the genes for important antigens will be transferred to harmless bacteria by simple laboratory tricks, thereby greatly facilitating vaccine production. It is most important that research into better, more effective, and safer vaccines proceeds concomitantly with that in fundamental or clinical immunology.

3

ANTIBODIES

CHRISTMAS EVE, 1891, was a dramatic turning point in the history of immunology. A little German girl was lying in von Bergmann's clinic in Berlin, suffering from diphtheria. She was entering a state of shock and seemed certain to succumb. The great German scientist, E. A. von Behring, decided to make her the first human guinea pig in a bold experiment—which saved her life and won him the first Nobel prize in medicine ten years later. Von Behring and Kitasato had discovered in 1890 that substances called *Antikörper* appeared in the bloodstream after infections, and were capable of neutralizing poisons in experimental animals. They had inoculated a sheep with diphtheria antigen, and now von Behring instructed Dr. Geissler to inject some of the sheep's serum into the dying child. In this way, they performed the first *passive immunization*, that is, the transfer of antibodies made by one animal or person to the bloodstream of another. Within hours the child began to revive. Her recovery signified a milestone—it was, in effect, the first occasion in which scientific medicine had contributed to the cure of an acute infectious disease.

In 1971, I had the great good fortune to be awarded the Emil von Behring Prize, which the Philipps University of Marburg instituted to perpetuate von Behring's memory. Many of the memorabilia of that first golden age of immunology are preserved in a beautiful reconstruction of von Behring's study housed within the Behringwerke, the large factory for vaccines, sera, and biologicals which he founded. Curiously, von Behring and his even more gifted compatriot Paul Ehrlich, were exactly the same age. They collaborated soon after the discovery of antibodies, but then had a great falling out. Ehrlich was excluded from the profits of the commercial venture which made von Behring a rich man, and after that they never again spoke to each other.

This chapter will be difficult, even tedious, in portions. Yet antibody structure provides so many clues to the wonders of the whole system that we must try to grasp it.

Nature of Antibodies

What, then, are antibodies? They are protein molecules present in the serum which have the capacity to unite with, and bind firmly to, an antigenic determinant on an antigen molecule. Moreover, they are highly specific molecules. For each antigen, there is a corresponding different antibody. As with locks and keys, only certain pairs fit. This is illustrated in Figure 3–1. Although the union between antigen and antibody is a firm one, it can be reversed by chemical processes such as heat, detergent, or acid treatment. The chief physical forces holding an antigen and an antibody together (hydrogen bonding, hydrophobic interactions, and van der Waals forces) are weaker than the so-called covalent interactions that hold different pieces of an individual molecule together. In fact, our purest preparations of antibodies are made by dissociation of antigen-antibody complexes.

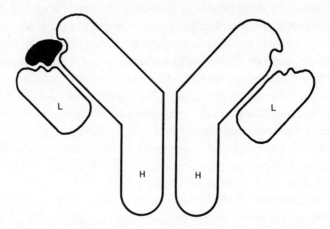

Figure 3–1. Specific complementarity between antigenic determinant and antibody-combining site. Note that both the light and heavy chains help to form the antibody-combining site.

As a rule antibodies are made only in response to the entry into the body of some antigen. In nature this will usually take place after infection with some foreign invader. In the laboratory and clinic it usually occurs after an injection of an antigen under the skin or into a muscle. Food contains many antigens but most of these are broken down into small, nonimmunogenic fragments by the digestive enzymes before being absorbed into the bloodstream. However, exceptions to this rule occur, and particularly in very young animals significant absorption of macromolecules from the gut has been observed. Food allergies can result from such exceptions.

Using the electron microscope, one can actually see antibody molecules, though their shapes are difficult to distinguish. However, we usually detect their presence and measure their concentration in the serum by much simpler means. These antibody *titration* methods depend on some observable interaction between antibody and antigen. For example, we can measure the capacity of a serum containing antibodies (*antiserum*) to form a precipitate with a solution of the antigen. The precipitation occurs because antibody molecules have two or more combining sites and antigens usually have more than one antigenic determinant. Thus a lattice structure is built up, as shown in Figure 3–2.

The precipitation reaction is of great historical interest, because it played a big role in making the study of antibody production a more quantitative science. In fact, the precipitin reaction is not altogether simple. If a mixture of antigen and antibody is made with a large excess of antigen and only a small amount of antibody, the statistics of collisions will be such that each of the (usually two) combining sites on the antibody molecules

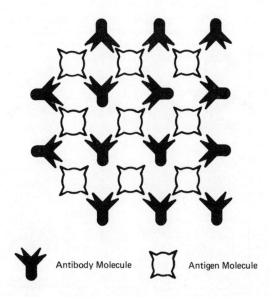

Antibody Molecule   Antigen Molecule

Figure 3–2. Lattice formation between antigen and antibody molecule. Note that the lattice can form only if both the antigen and the antibody have more than one binding site.

will attach to antigen molecules that, even though they possess
available sites, have no other antibody molecules attached to
them. Thus no lattice forms. At the other extreme, if there are
far more antibody than antigen molecules in the reaction mixture, all the antigenic determinants on a given antigen molecule
will rapidly become occupied by one of the teeming crowd of
antibody molecules, resulting in no free sites for possible bridge-
building to other antigen molecules. In the intermediate situation, cross-linking of antigen molecules by antibody molecules
depends on their relative concentrations. This results in a characteristic curve describing the precipitation reaction, as shown
in Figure 3–3. Maximal precipitation occurs at the *zone of
equivalence*, where the number of antigen molecules equals the

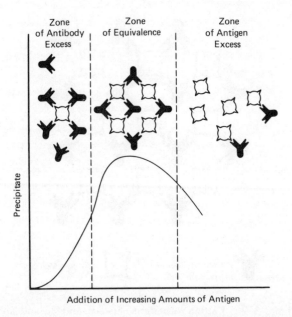

Figure 3–3.   Precipitin curve describing quantitative features of antigen-antibody union.

number of antibody molecules. At higher or lower concentrations, some soluble complexes will be present. As the antigen-antibody reaction is reversible, there will always be a dynamic equilibrium situation. For most practical purposes, however, the bias is towards relatively stable binding. By exposing antisera to antigens bound to a solid phase (such as a glass bead), one can absorb out essentially all of the specific antibodies from a serum sample with relatively little trouble. One can then elute off the antibodies from the immunoabsorbent, providing relatively pure antibodies.

If the antigen is a preparation of whole bacteria, the lattice formed results in very large particles readily seen with the naked eye. Such lattices are called *agglutinates*. Similarly, antibodies made against foreign cells such as red blood corpuscles can cause visible agglutination of the cell antigen. These reactions are widely used by immunologists who can thus measure the concentration of antibodies in a serum very quickly and without expensive equipment. Other antibody measurement procedures depend on the antibody's interfering with some vital function of the antigen. For example, one can assess how many virus particles can be rendered noninfectious, or how many enzyme molecules nonactive, by a sample of serum. There are also many other ways in which antibody molecules manifest their presence to the investigator, but they all depend on the same property— the capacity of the combining site to form a firm union with an antigenic determinant.

The Chemical Structure of Antibodies

Considering the large size of the antibody molecule, which contains 1300 amino-acid building blocks on the average, and some of the difficulties in obtaining pure antibodies, which I shall detail, the amount we know about antibody structure is little short of astonishing, and is a tribute both to the scientists who have labored over the problem these last 20 years, and to the elegance and complexity of the techniques which we now possess to study protein structure. Mammals make five different chemical types of antibodies which play distinct physiological roles, but most of our structural knowledge comes from one type, IgG, which I shall now describe. Since the very early days of blood analysis, serum proteins were broken up into *albumins* (egg white-like proteins) and *globulins* (more or less all the rest). All antibodies, normal and abnormal, are known generically as immunoglobulins, or simply Ig. The most abundant chemical type of antibody in man is known as IgG. The older phrase, "gamma globulin," is still used to describe serum preparations rich in IgG, but these are prepared by rather simple fractionation methods which leave in them significant numbers of other immunoglobulins and, indeed, quite different proteins. IgG has a molecular weight of about 160,000 and contains not only the amino acids, which we shall discuss in some detail, but also a small amount of carbohydrate; the latter is important, but it does not concern the combining specificity of the molecule.

Like many proteins, IgG is really a hybrid molecule, consisting in fact of four separate molecules or *polypeptide chains*. Two of these have about 440 amino acids each, and are called heavy chains; two possess 220 amino acids and are called light chains. In any one IgG molecule, the two heavy chains are always identical to each other, as are the two light chains. The four chains are bound to one another both by the strong chemical covalent bond, known as a disulfide bridge, and by weaker forces such as hydrogen bonding. A disulfide bridge occurs when two molecules of the amino acid cysteine are brought together, and the adjacent -SH groups are oxidized into an -S-S- bridge.

There are various ways of depicting IgG structure schematically, and one of these is given in Figure 3–4. This two-

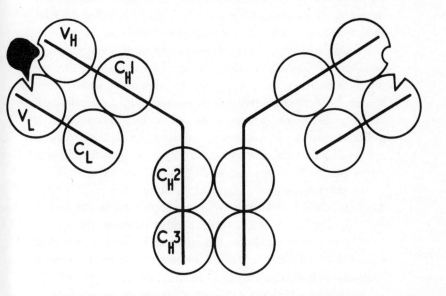

Figure 3–4. Schematic view of an IgG molecule. This simplified diagram shows that each chain is composed of "domains" which have a basically similar structure.

dimensional representation shows us that each light chain has two regions or *domains* that are rather similar to each other, while each heavy chain has four domains, each similar to the others and also to those of the light chain. A prominent feature of each domain is a loop of about 60 amino acids arising from an *intrachain disulfide bond*. The figure further shows that the *antibody-combining site* is formed jointly by the light and heavy chains, and that the molecule is bilaterally symmetrical, each molecule having two absolutely identical combining sites. The molecule has a handle (known as the Fc portion) and two identical arms (known as the Fab portions) thus forming the shape of a Y. In fact, it is known to be rather flexible at the hinge region of the Y. To anticipate a little, each light chain consists of one V, or variable domain, and one C, or constant domain, and each heavy chain of one V and three C domains.

Though accurate as far as it goes, Figure 3–4 is not meant to be taken too literally. In three-dimensional terms, proteins are not like necklaces, linear strings of the component amino acids. Rather, they are intricately shaped precision tools, the individual amino acids folding to make a complex sculptural contour. It is this final shape which confers on a protein the capacity to interact specifically with another protein, as in a three-dimensional jigsaw puzzle. Yet even this analogy oversimplifies matters, as, unlike intricately chiseled pieces of wood, proteins are not rigid. They can change their shape when they meet another molecule, and this very change might reveal another new site with special combining properties. Thus, the molecule is more than a tool; it is in fact a machine. When a protein is composed of more than one polypeptide chain, as in the case of antibodies, the various chains intertwine with each other, heavy and light chains together forming a combining site.

An elegant technique, known as X-ray crystallography, can give us the structure of proteins in the manner most nearly approximating three-dimensional sculpture. Under the best circumstances, the technique can depict the size, shape, and relative location of each atom of the molecule. X-ray crystallographers have built large-scale models of the molecules they are investigating, and have wandered around them for many hours studying the subtlety of their construction. Various simpler representations of the structure have included the more conventional wire models, or even two-dimensional linear projections which serve as a convenient shorthand in publications. Crystals of both Fab and Fc portions of IgG have been subjected to intensive study over the last few years, and have revealed much about the antibody-combining site, which covers an appreciable area on the surface of the molecule. While only about 20 of the 440 amino acids of one Fab are actual contact residues in the site, as many as 70 influence the shape of the site by pushing and pulling the amino acids in various ways. X-ray crystallography has also confirmed most of the features of the domain model (Figure 3–4), which was presented before the X-ray data came to hand.

Variability of Combining Sites

When a mother drives to school on an afternoon to pick up her son, she may be confronted with dozens or even hundreds of children, playing in the schoolyard, all having much the same shapes and sizes. Yet, unerringly and without conscious effort, she picks out the correct child, and would do so even if there were 100,000 to choose from. What characteristic of her Johnny allows her to do this? Undoubtedly, the most important feature is his face. We have no trouble in noting quite minor differences in the sizes and shapes of people's noses, mouths, eyes—and somehow our brains integrate these into a total visual picture of a face which is unmistakable. Moreover, we know that though the allowable variation in the sizes of noses or jaws, for example, is quite small, the total number of obviously different faces is huge—certainly in the millions. So it is with antibodies, and the distinctive "face" of the antibody molecule is the combining site. Just like the schoolchildren, all IgG molecules have the same shape, and the two combining sites have much the same size. Yet a seemingly endless variety of detailed patterns exists. Thus an antigen has no more trouble "recognizing" and linking with its relevant antibody than does the mother in finding Johnny. The combining site is therefore the key to the exquisite specificity and unique variability of antibodies.

A further look at our model (Figure 3–4) will show how cunningly nature has designed this vital active region of the antibody molecule. It is a region to which *both* of the component chains contribute. Returning to our "face" analogy, we will see how much extra variability this can confer on the shape of the site. Suppose we come to a small Polynesian island where the natives are rather inbred. Many of the individuals look alike, and we may occasionally have trouble telling them apart. Imbued with a missionary zeal, we are determined to make the population monogamous. Accordingly, we produce a great many handcuffs and proceed to bind each woman to one man. Of course, our plan is doomed to failure, but we are soon struck by an unexpected "fringe benefit." Identification has become easier! When we have trouble telling two of the men apart, we simply look at their corresponding women and this gives us an extra way of discriminating between them. The pair has a greater individuality than each partner. Moreover, if there had been 100 men and 100 women on the island, we could have constructed 10,000 different handcuffed pairs. So it is with the globulin chains. For example, if the body knows how to make 1,000 different varieties of both light and heavy chains, a million different antibody types could result. (The importance of this will emerge more fully in Chapter 4.)

Amino-acid Sequence Studies on Immunoglobulin Chains

What is the chemical basis on which the variation in the "face" of the antibody, the combining site, rests? For a long time this was uncertain. Early theories of antibody specificity assumed that the basic stuff of a globulin molecule was like a soft piece of wax, formless and malleable, and capable of being pressed or molded into a variety of shapes by the antigen. However, modern studies have shown quite clearly that antibodies differ in *chemical composition* as well as in the shape of the combining site.

We have already learned that antibodies are proteins and are made up of amino-acid building blocks. There are 20 different kinds of amino acids, which we can think of as corresponding to the 26 letters of the alphabet. Out of 26 letters, we can construct the English language. I never cease to wonder at the fact that the very considerable differences between, say, William Shakespeare and Saul Bellow can all be described in terms of the different ways that they have used these 26 building blocks. Similarly, the difference between the blood pigment of a keyhole limpet and the insulin of a man can be described in terms of the 20 letters of the language of proteins. It is simply a question of the number and sequential arrangement of the amino acids which constitute the protein concerned.

If you are a discerning reader you will object: "But this analogy is ridiculous! A page of writing is really only a one-dimensional string of symbols and spaces, whereas, clearly, a protein must be a three-dimensional entity capable of contorting into a variety of shapes." Amazingly enough, your objection is not valid. It has been shown time and again that given a particular sequence of amino acids, a protein will spontaneously assume a particular shape. The three-dimensional or "tertiary" structure is already inherent in the "primary" sequence of amino acids. A discussion of how this comes about would take us far afield into the realm of theoretical chemistry. Therefore, let us accept the finding as one of the secrets of life and see how it affects the antibody problem.

We now know the full amino-acid sequence of quite a few immunoglobulin light and heavy chains. Yet, right throughout the 1950s and halfway through the 1960s, the vital tool of amino-acid sequence analysis could not be applied to the antibody problem. The reason was simple. Sequence analysis of proteins requires substantial amounts of very pure protein. But even when pure antigens are used to immunize animals, the antibody synthesized as a result is far from pure. First, several or all of the different classes are made, and IgG possesses subclasses as well. Second, different cells will recognize and react to different portions of the antigenic mosaic, and the result is a heterogeneous population of antibody molecules. It is certainly no use trying to sequence a mishmash of many proteins.

A fortunate feature of an unfortunate event has come to our rescue. Occasionally, in both mice and men, an antibody-forming cell turns cancerous and overgrows wildly. As a result, vast quantities of its product are made and enter the bloodstream. It is a rule of the immune system (see Chapter 5) that one cell makes only one antibody, and so the product of the cancer is a pure immunoglobulin, ideal for sequence studies. Later research has also revealed that certain carbohydrate antigens could evoke the formation of very pure antibodies in a proportion of the rabbits into which they were injected.

If we look at the amino-acid sequence of three different light chains, say, from three individuals each with a different tumor, we find a strange state of affairs. The sequence can be symbolized by three words:

SPEEDING
SPENDING
SCOLDING

When we write these three words immediately below each other, we notice several things. First of all, each word can be broken into a variable region and a constant region. The last four letters are always DING—this is the constant region of our set of words. The first four letters constitute a variable region. Note that the constant region and variable region are of exactly equal length. Look a little more closely and you will see that a portion of the variable region is invariant. At position 1, each word possesses the letter S. Finally, note that at one of the other positions (position 4), there are three alternative letters, but at positions 2 and 3 there are only two alternative letters. This is a fair approximation of the way in which evolution has designed antibody chains.

The human immunoglobulin light chain is more complex than any of our words. In fact, it contains 220 letters rather than 8. However, the whole chain is divisible into two halves. One half, containing 110 amino acids, is of constant structure, like the DING portion of our three words. The other half, also containing 110 amino acids, is highly variable, and on this variability rests the great diversity of antibody combining sites. However, not each of the 110 positions in this variable segment is in fact variant. Over half the positions are like the S in position 1 of our words; that is, the same amino acid appears in all the different light chains studied so far at those particular positions. At the other positions in the stretch from 1 to 110, variations occur. At some of these, as in positions 2 and 3 of our model word, only two alternatives have been noted so far. At others, the variation is less restrictive. Clearly, the total number of different types of light chains that can be constructed is immense. The amino acids in the variable domain that are invariant are known as framework residues. They are needed to give the domain its overall shape. If, instead of three words, we had placed 20 homologous molecules under one another, we would have noted that variation showed up much more frequently over certain particular short stretches of the molecule than at others. Correlation of amino acid sequence and X-ray crystallographic data has shown that the amino acids of these hypervariable stretches in fact poke and fold their way into the combining site. Though exploration of the structure of the heavy chain is not yet as extensive, it is clear that the above basic rules apply. Instead of two domains, as in the light chain, there are four domains. Only one of these at one end of the molecule (the so-called N-terminal) is variable between antibodies, and it has hypervariable stretches contributing to the combining site. The three constant domains show homologies to one another and also to the C domains of light chains.

Immunoglobulin Classes, Subclasses, and Subgroups

If the above description has seemed a little complex, let me try the reader's patience still further and say that it is, in fact, an oversimplification. We have referred already to the five different chemical kinds of antibodies. Each of these possesses a heavy chain with its own particular type of constant region, different in sequence from the constant region of IgG. Each of these five chains is named by a Greek letter: gamma (γ), mu (μ), alpha (α), epsilon (ϵ), and delta (δ). In man, the γ chains fall into four subclasses (γ_1, γ_2, γ_3 and γ_4) which more resemble one another than any of the other classes, yet are sufficiently different from one another for us to realize they are the products of separate genes. Subclasses of the other classes are still being discovered. There may well be 12 or more classes and subclasses in all. There are also two kinds of light chains, bearing the Greek letters kappa (κ) and lambda (λ), either of which can come into combination with any of the heavy chains. The five major classes of Ig are named for their heavy chains, thus IgG, IgM, IgA, IgE, and IgD. It is the nature of the heavy chain which confers on the molecule its overall biological properties (as opposed to its combining specificity, which follows the same rules for all the classes). The shorthand IgG does not, however, tell us whether a molecule consists of two κ and two γ_1 chains, or perhaps of two λ and two γ_3 chains. If there are, say, a dozen subclasses of heavy chains altogether, there will be 24 chemically different types of antibodies as far as the *constant* portion of the molecule is concerned. Of course, this is a small number when compared with the millions or billions of different sorts of combining sites, but as each animal in a species exhibits *all* of the chemical classes (unless suffering from some deficiency disease), it does represent a substantial complexity for immunological studies.

So much for the different kinds of constant regions. What of the variable regions? The first point is that there are three fundamental sorts of variable regions, namely those of κ chains, those of λ chains, and those of heavy chains, known respectively as V_κ, V_λ, and V_H. The fact that the different classes of heavy chains share the one overall sort of V region is surprising and unique, and will be discussed in Chapter 5.

For each of these three types of V regions, one can perform sequence analysis of a number of different antibodies. When, for example, the sequences of 20 different V_κ regions are determined, and the alphabetical representations are linked up one underneath the other, it is at once apparent that some of the sequences, though variant, are more like one another than others. In other words, the sequences can be arranged into subgroups. For example, there are three major subgroups of V_κ in the mouse. Some scientists believe that the subgroups can be further divided into sub-subgroups. This is not an arcane and pointless game, but is essential for our understanding of the nature of antibody diversity, as we shall see in Chapter 5. For the moment, the key point to remember is that each subgroup must be coded by a different gene.

Allotypy and Idiotypy

Antibodies, like other proteins, can function as antigens. One can thus prepare anti-antibodies. This important fact will raise its head several times. In our consideration of the structure of antibodies, the importance of anti-antibodies lies in the fact that they have allowed us to discover two further ways of approaching antibody diversity, namely allotypy and idiotypy. Allotypy means that different individuals of a species may make very slightly different chemical kinds of antibodies. (Technically speaking, the antibody genes are polymorphic in that species.)

This is because one or more of the amino acids in a particular constant region, or in a framework residue of a variable region, differs genetically. One can think of allotypes of immunoglobulins as somewhat analogous to blood groups among red cells. One person possesses one group, another a different set. Idiotypy means that the uniqueness of the combining site of a particular, pure antibody can be recognized by the immune system, and one can make antibodies which will react with the antibody-combining site yet not with other immunoglobulins of that class, even in the same individual. We shall encounter idiotypy again in Chapter 10.

Biological Functions of Antibody Classes

If all the antibody classes possess combining sites of the same general design, why did nature go to the trouble of devising so many different classes? The reason is that each heavy chain class, or more precisely each Fc handle portion of immunoglobulin, possesses its own set of very special characteristics, which confer certain biological properties on the molecule, differing from class to class.

IgG is the most abundant class, the "standard" antibody. It is very good at neutralizing toxins, and it crosses the placenta readily, thereby conferring protection against common diseases from mother to baby. For reasons to be discussed, the body can produce IgG of a very high combining strength or affinity for antigen.

IgM is the next most abundant immunoglobulin and is probably the most ancient form. It originally derived its name from its size—a macroglobulin—or very large molecule of molecular weight 900,000. It consists of no fewer than 20 chains, 10 heavy and 10 light, giving it 10 combining sites, and it also possesses more carbohydrate than IgG. Even IgM of a relatively low affinity can attach very efficiently to a bacterium or other antigen with multiple antigenic determinants (multivalent antigen) because it can use its multiple combining sites in combinatorial fashion to gain a firmer grip on the antigen. Technically, we say that even *low affinity* antibodies can be of *high avidity* because of this trick. IgM is the first class of antibody to be made by very young animals, and it is also the first to appear in time after an immunization of adults—sensitive techniques picking up its presence already 36 to 48 hours after an antigen injection. These observations, taken together, suggest that IgM is a kind of "panic button" antibody, IgG representing a later evolutionary refinement. A four-chain variant of IgM (two heavy and two light chains) exists on the surface of lymphocytes, to be described in Chapters 4 and 5.

IgA is nature's antiseptic ointment. Also known as secretory immunoglobulin, it has the special property of crossing cell barriers easily and it appears in high concentration in secretions such as tears, saliva, nasal, bronchial, or gut mucus, and even breast milk. It serves a valuable function in repelling microbial invasion via the various linings and openings of the body. Most IgA is the same size as IgG, but some molecules exist as larger polymers.

IgE will be described in detail in Chapter 18. It is the prime antibody involved in allergies. We can only speculate about its true physiological role, as obviously allergy is a nuisance and not a help to the body. Perhaps the allergic reaction is an exaggerated form of a response which, if quite mild, aids the inflammatory process to get rid of foreign material which floats into the nose or respiratory tract. IgE is a four-chain polymer.

IgD is present in only trace amounts in human serum, and cannot be detected at all in the serum of the mouse. However, like IgM, it is present in large quantities as a receptor on the surface of lymphocytes, where its role remains somewhat mysterious. We shall encounter it again in the next two chapters.

Cross-reactions among Antibodies

So far we have been talking as though the correlation between an antigenic determinant and the corresponding antibody combining site were absolute. However, this is not the case. Every self-respecting burglar knows that more than one key can open a lock. Similarly, for every given antigenic determinant, the body can construct a variety of antibody combining sites—some of which fit almost perfectly, and others which barely fit at all. This is shown in Figure 3–5, although we must remember that we should think in three dimensions, not two. Moreover, an antibody molecule made following the injection of one antigen can frequently combine with a second antigen of a related or similar shape, though the fit will not be quite as good. In other words, the antibody cross-reacts with the second antigen. This concept of cross-reactivity is important for immunological theory. The number of antigenic determinants in the universe, including both

Native Antigen

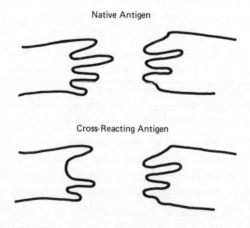

Cross-Reacting Antigen

Figure 3–5.   Cross-reactivity among antigens.

naturally occurring organic molecules plus the whole gamut of synthetic compounds, is perhaps not infinite but is certainly enormously large. The number of different antibody combining sites which an animal can make is also large, but is unlikely to exceed 10 million or 100 million. It is simply because the fit between antigens and antibodies need not be perfect (just as an incomplete key may open a lock) that the body can turn out antibodies against virtually anything. On its bountiful key ring the body will find at least one key which fits sufficiently well to open any lock. Here is your first clue to the way the immune system does its job without breaking genetic laws!

How Antibodies Work

We have referred above to the power of antibodies to kill bacteria and to perform other useful tasks. Frequently, however, antibodies can do their job only in collaboration with other bodily defense mechanisms. In the pre-antibiotic era, every large hospital had many beds filled with patients suffering from pneumonia. Experienced physicians could usually see the crisis of each sufferer approaching. For seven days or so, the patient grew progressively worse. Frequently he died, but in other cases his symptoms would abate with dramatic suddenness, and within hours he would be out of danger. By microscopic study of the lungs we can determine what was going on. As the deadly pneumonia-causers, the pneumococci, grew inside the lung spaces, or alveoli, they caused inflammation. Scavenger cells of various sorts were sent scurrying after the bacteria. At first, these seemed remarkably inefficient. With great motility and speed they attempted to corner their prey, but somehow most of the cocci got away. In fact, they thrived and multiplied to such an extent that whole lobes of the lung were converted to a soggy,

inflamed mess. Then, quite suddenly, the enemy became de-
moralized and seemingly gave up the struggle. This corre-
sponded with the time of the crisis. From this point on, if the
patient were fortunate enough to reach it, the scavenger cells
began to gobble up the bacteria most effectively and very soon
carried the day. What was responsible? In this case, it was a
phenomenon known as *opsonization*. The antipneumococcal
antibodies were the secret weapon, and their appearance in the
bloodstream at the time of crisis marked the turning point. For
some reason, scavenger cells are very poor at eating bacteria
raw. However, when the microbes are coated or "buttered" with
antibodies stuck onto their surfaces they become much more
palatable to the scavenger cells which then literally stuff themselves full and digest the meal. The great English bacteriologist,
Almroth Wright, popularized the word "opsonin" to describe
the antibody molecules which were effective in this way. The
concept seemed to tickle the fancy of George Bernard Shaw,
who referred to it in *The Doctor's Dilemma*. In this case, the
opsonic antibodies could not kill the pneumococci by themselves, and neither could the scavenger cells, but both in combination were magically effective.

Another even more complex example of how antibodies work
is the way they kill bacteria. In normal blood serum there exists
a group of proteins known collectively as the complement system. This system can be thought of as a sheathed dagger. Circulating around the body, it is quite harmless. However, when
an antibody molecule meets an antigen, for example, on the surface of a bacterium, the antigen-antibody complex tends to at-
tract and "fix" some of the complement components. This fixation
of complement leads to a violent and complex chain reaction,
involving no fewer than nine well-studied proteins, leading
finally to the activation of powerful destructive enzymes. At the
site of the antigen-antibody-complement union, a stiletto-like
hole is punched into the bacterial wall and the bacterium bursts,
or "lyses." IgM is several hundred times more efficient than IgG

in this regard, probably because of its special ability to cause complement fixation. The early appearance of IgM thus helps greatly in serious infections.

A third way in which antibodies work is by covering up some vital structural component of a microbe. For example, some viruses have elaborate structures on their surfaces for attaching themselves onto a host cell and penetrating it. Antibodies directed against these components may be quite incapable of killing the virus directly. Yet the end result is just as deleterious because the vital anchoring mechanism of the virus is all glued up. If it cannot parasitize the cell, the virus cannot grow, and if it cannot grow, it cannot invade and kill the host. There are many other ways in which the tiny, and in themselves innocuous, antibody molecules can aid the body. Occasionally, however, the process boomerangs and antibodies actually cause disease. How this comes about will be discussed in Chapters 18 and 19.

4

IMMUNOCYTE CELLS

THE RECOGNITION of foreignness and its eventual conquest by the immune system are a special example of warfare. If an army is to engage in jungle warfare, the soldiers will be trained to deal with the enemy in a number of different ways. Among other things, the soldiers will learn how to shoot from a distance and also how to engage in man-to-man combat. This is similar to the two basic ways in which lymphocytes are trained by evolution to react to invaders which attack the body. So far we have discussed mainly the shooting war—the production by stimulated lymphocytes and their progeny of antibodies which travel in the bloodstream and, like bullets, act on the antigenic particle or molecules at some distance from their source of origin. This broad aspect of the defense system is described as *humoral immunity*, a humoral substance being anything which is synthesized in one place and travels through the circulation to exert an action at another place in the body. Now we must turn our attention to the other chief division of immunology, namely, cellular immunity. This is a process whereby immunologically active lymphocytes actually make contact with foreign antigens and exert a local, direct killing action.

The two great divisions of the immune response, cellular immunity and humoral immunity, depend on two quite different families or sets of lymphocytes respectively termed T and B cells for short. Having looked at antigens and antibodies, we must now focus the spotlight on these cells, the third group of actors in our drama. The existence of cellular immunity was known as a distinct immunological entity well before T and B cells were discovered. Therefore, before describing these so-called *immunocytes* (a generic term for all the lymphocytes and their progeny) in detail, we should look at what cellular immunity or cell-mediated immunity really is.

A good example of a cellular immune phenomenon is the tuberculin reaction. Most nurses and medical students will know this reaction, which is essentially a test to see whether a person has ever been infected with tuberculosis. The test is performed as follows. A purified protein called tuberculin, derived from tubercle bacteria, is injected into the skin of the forearm. In a person who has never had even a touch of tuberculosis, or BCG vaccination, nothing happens. There is no local reaction to the injection, and as tuberculin by itself is not an immunogenic form of antigen, the person does not become immunized. Now there are many people in the community who contract tuberculosis but conquer it before any damage is done. In fact, they usually do not even know that they have had it. If such a person is given tuberculin into the skin, a characteristic sequence of events follows. Nothing is observed for several hours. Gradually, however, a little hard lump appears in the skin. In about 48 hours it reaches maximum size and is red and inflamed; then it slowly fades away over the next few days. A typical reaction will be about half an inch in diameter and about a tenth of an inch raised from the surface, but strongly positive reactions can be much bigger and angrier. A person who reacts thus to the injection is termed tuberculin positive. Usually an attack of tuberculosis, however mild and transient, will make a person tuberculin positive for life. It is a good diagnostic test for evidence of past or present tuberculosis infection, unless, of course, the person has been vaccinated with BCG, which turns on cell-mediated immunity and also makes the test positive.

Naturally, experimentation on the nature of this little lump is very limited in the human. Fortunately, guinea pigs behave in a basically similar manner and so we have a detailed picture of what is involved. Microscopic study of a positive reaction reveals that the deeper layers of the skin are infiltrated with large numbers of lymphocytes and monocytes, or scavenger white blood cells. Because of the fact that the reaction is much slower to develop than allergic reactions, this acquired special sensitivity to tuberculin as a result of prior antigenic stimulation by living tubercle bacilli is termed an example of *delayed hypersensitivity*.

Serum Antibodies Not Involved in Delayed Hypersensitivity

Delayed hypersensitivity, an example of a cellular immune phenomenon, would not be of much interest to us if it were simply a handy diagnostic test. It is important to remember that similar lymphocyte and monocyte infiltrations will also be occurring around the site of multiplication of the living tubercle bacteria in the lung of a TB sufferer. Still more vital to us is the knowledge that basically similar processes are at work when an organ graft is being rejected by the body. Is delayed hypersensitivity simply due to some form of serum antibody? For an answer to this question we must consult an experiment depicted in Figure 4–1. If one takes a tuberculin-positive guinea pig and injects large quantities of its serum, with whatever antibodies it contains, into a normal, tuberculin-negative guinea pig, a subsequent test of the recipient shows that it is still tuberculin nega-

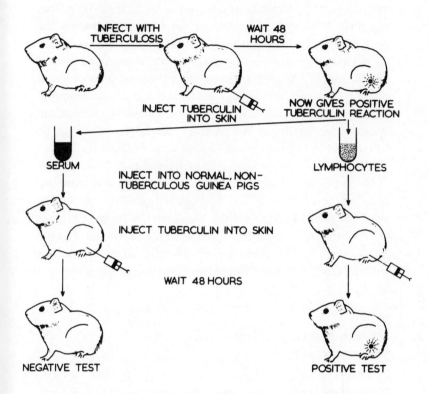

Figure 4–1. The transfer of delayed hypersensitivity.

tive. If the reaction had been due to circulating antibodies, these would have been present in the recipient guinea pig and should have conferred on it a passive immunity. If, instead of transferring serum, one takes a suspension of lymphocytes either from the blood or from a lymphoid organ and injects these into the recipient guinea pig, a different result is observed. The guinea pig now gives a positive reaction. It will continue to be tuberculin positive for as long as the foreign lymphocytes survive in it. This shows that the delayed hypersensitivity reaction depends on the activity of lymphocyte cells rather than on circulating antibodies. The procedure of transferring an immune state from one animal to another by means of lymphocyte suspensions has been widely used in research. It is called *adoptive immunization*. In contrast, the transfer of serum antibodies is called *passive immunization*. Delayed hypersensitivity, capacity to react to organ grafts, and immunological memory can all be conferred by adoptive immunization but not by passive immunization. Antitoxic immunity, as von Behring showed in 1891, can be transferred by passive immunization and as we shall see, so can allergic or *immediate hypersensitivity* reactions.

In the mouse, a great deal of work has been done on adoptive transfers of all kinds of immunological reactions, and in this species our capacity to separate T and B cells from each other is greatest. Experiments have proven conclusively that it is the T cell which is responsible for cell-mediated immunity. But, as we shall see, T cells have many other intriguing jobs to do!

Rejection of Organ Grafts as a Cellular Immune Reaction

If one observes the course of events occurring in a skin graft taken from one individual and placed in a wound on another individual, the similarities to a tuberculin reaction are striking. There is no immediate reaction. In fact, the graft heals into place just as well as if it had been taken from a different part of the recipient's own body. As soon as healing has taken place, antigens leak from the graft. They set up a state of cellular immunity in the host. As a result, lymphocytes and monocytes invade the graft. It soon turns red and swollen, then black, and within seven to ten days of the initial operation, it drops off. Microscopic sections of the skin during the rejection phase will show massive infiltration of the deep layers with host cells. Once the graft has been thrown off, the host animal remains immune for long periods. It manifests its cellular immune state just as does the patient recovered from tuberculosis. In other words, antigenic extracts prepared from the skin of the original donor can be injected into the immune animal, and lumps just like those of a tuberculin reaction will be raised. Moreover, the once-grafted animal will, for the rest of its life, retain the capacity to reject a second graft from the same donor in accelerated fashion.

You will have realized by now that things in immunology are rarely quite straightforward. For a long time it was thought that the rejection of organ grafts was due wholly and solely to cellular immune phenomena. Now we know that there are circumstances in which serum antibodies to graft antigens can contribute damage. (We will examine this when we discuss kidney transplantation in man.) It is still true, however, that the chief factor in immunological graft rejection is a phenomenon akin to delayed hypersensitivity. We must now look more closely at the various steps involved in this reaction to a graft.

Hierarchies of Immunocytes

We can look at lymphocytes in either the optical or the electron microscope and note their overall similarity. They are really very unremarkable kinds of cells, with little cytoplasm and apparently not much action going on inside them. This apparent uniformity is an utter deception, and failure to realize the great functional heterogeneity amongst similar looking lymphocytes held back immunology for decades. Now, through intensive research over the last few years, we can classify lymphocytes into an orderly, though surely not yet complete, scheme.

The first point to grasp is that there are basically three hierarchies to be considered in each of the two lymphocyte families. These can be summarized by the words *genesis*, *watchfulness*, *action*.

Just as children are quite obviously human before they can do any useful task, so cells may look like lymphocytes but not yet be ready to react with antigens. In fact, there is a process of genesis of lymphocytes, also termed lymphoneogenesis, about which a lot is known; this will be discussed in Chapter 8. For the purposes of the present analysis, suffice it to say that there exist cells which look like lymphocytes, but which actually represent "pre-B" and "pre-T" cells. They are undergoing a maturation phase. They will soon be ready to act as the body's policemen but have not yet finished their schooling.

Once lymphocytes, be they T cells or B cells, are mature, they wander around the body and, in their *watchfulness*, resemble policemen on the beat. While all is quiet they do little except travel around. Most of the lymphocytes of the body of an adult animal or person are in this hierarchy. They are not dividing, they are not secreting antibody molecules, they are not mounting a cell-mediated attack; they are simply watching and waiting for an antigen to come along.

When an antigen enters the body, some of the lymphocytes are triggered into *action*. Their metabolic processes speed up. They enlarge and begin to multiply. These activated immunocytes constitute the third hierarchy of so-called immunological effector cells. They secrete antibodies if they are B cells or attack the antigenic cell or microbe if they are T cells. Frequently, their activated state can be guessed at by the greater amount of activity in the cytoplasm shown up by certain stains in the ordinary microscope. But some effector cells really look virtually indistinguishable from their ancestors, the watchful cells, and their true nature is revealed only by functional tests. At the other extreme, some progeny of B lymphocytes develop a very elaborate cytoplasmic machinery for the large-scale secretion of antibodies, and thereby develop a characteristic shape and appearance. These are called plasma cells. We shall meet them in detail in Chapter 13.

Unfortunately, when the terms T and B cells are used in an unqualified fashion, it is frequently not clear to which of these three hierarchies the author is referring. Rather, the terms are used in their generic sense to describe one of the two great families of cells. An older classification of lymphocytes was into large, medium, and small, and this simple description is still in use in routine clinical hematology. However, such grouping conveys limited information. It does not discriminate between T and B cells. It is true that most mature T and B cells in the watchful state are small, nondividing cells, but so are some pre-B and pre-T cells as well as some active effector cells of both families. Conversely, the cells that are large and rapidly dividing, or medium and relatively slowly dividing, may be either in the genesis compartment, in the process of making T or B cells, or in the action hierarchy, engaged in enlarging the family of effector cells. Classification of human lymphocytes by size alone will continue for some time because it is not practicable to perform on every routine blood smear the more elaborate tests needed to subclassify them.

The Concept of Lymphocyte Receptors for Antigen

The next major facet of immunocyte functioning to be understood is how the watchful T or B lymphocyte actually knows that an antigen is around and that it must spring into action. This key question in cellular immunology will concern us again and again, and at this stage I want to introduce the concept of *lymphocyte receptors* for antigen, which will become much clearer in the next chapter.

Lymphocytes know that antigen is in their environment because, in their mature, watchful state, they possess molecules on their surface (as an integral part of the outer membrane or skin of the cell) which have the capacity to recognize and react with antigen. Activation or triggering of the lymphocyte is a consequence of a union of an antigen molecule with a cell surface receptor for that antigen. Here, then, is your second clue to nature's strategy in the design of the immune system.

The receptor on the watchful B cell's surface is itself an antibody. B cells first emerging from the B lymphocyte "school" (Chapter 8) have receptors of the IgM class only. A proportion later also display IgD. A typical B lymphocyte has 100,000 Ig molecules on its surface.

The problem of the receptor for antigen on the T cell has been much more controversial but now appears to be nearing resolution. It is certain that V_H domains are involved, in other words that the T cell receptor possesses a heavy chain with a V region like the V regions of regular immunoglobulin. The C regions are different, however, and the heavy chain can be regarded as a new class perhaps most nearly resembling a μ chain. Light chains have been detected on the T cell surface by some authors but not by others. The total number of antigen receptors is much smaller—probably 10,000 per cell or less. There is something strange about the recognition properties of T cells; they seem to react best to foreign molecules presented to the T cell in association with certain other antigens important in organ transplantation. T cells as a whole display an extraordinary capacity to react to transplant antigens from other individuals in the same species. These facts will seem mysterious to the reader but will become clearer later. Their implication may be that the T cell possesses a second set of (nonimmunoglobulin-like) receptors with reactivity against certain tissue antigens.

These various receptors for antigen are acquired during lymphoneogenesis and, in the case of the B cell, are sometimes lost after activation of the cell into an antibody-producing effector immunocyte (plasma cell).

Further T Cell Functions and Subsets

Receptors for antigens are by no means the only interesting proteins that appear on the lymphocyte surface. In fact, there are a number of others, the function of which is not understood, but which have caused great recent excitement in immunology research circles. These are surface molecules which are characteristic of T lymphocytes (allowing these to be distinguished from B lymphocytes with certainty) and other molecules which occur on some but not all T cells, alerting us to the fact that T cells fall into subsets.

In the mouse, these molecules as a class have been identified not by their physical or chemical properties but by their antigenic characteristics. They are members of the class of *lymphocyte differentiation antigens*. The two most important groups are the Thy–1 or theta (θ) antigen, characteristic of *all* members of the T cell family; and the Ly antigens, which have been crucial in breaking T cells into subsets. Of the Ly antigens, the most important are Ly 1, 2, and 3. Cells possessing Ly 1 but not 2 and 3 belong to the "helper" subset of T cells, and those positive for the Ly 2 and 3 antigens to the "killer/suppressor" subset, the functions of which I shall now describe.

So far in our consideration of T cells, we have concentrated on two phenomena: delayed hypersensitivity, which depends on activated T cells meeting antigen and secreting factors which promote inflammation; and graft rejection, which depends on the direct cytotoxic killing of grafted cells by activated T cells. We now have fairly good quantitative methods for measuring the former activity in a population of T lymphocytes isolated in a test tube, and excellent quantitative measures of the latter killer phenomenon. Now we must meet some of the subtler functions of antigenically activated T effector cells, namely as regulators of B cell function.

When I said in the last section that lymphocytes get triggered
as a result of a union between lymphocyte surface receptors and
antigens, the statement was correct but also very incomplete. In
fact, triggering is by no means the inevitable result of such a
meeting. In many cases, the activation must be *helped* in ways
we do not yet understand by the interactive participation of a
special subset of T cells, the helper T cells. These possess the
Ly 1 antigen but not the Ly 2, 3 and are therefore termed Ly
1^+, 2^-, 3^-. The cells responsible for transferring delayed hypersensitivity from one mouse to another are also Ly 1^+, 2^-, 3^-.

While the importance of helper T cells has been known for
nearly a decade, a second type of regulatory T cell of great
significance has been discovered more recently. This is the *suppressor T cell*. When it is activated by antigen, it in some way
hampers the activation of B lymphocytes. It thus suppresses
antibody formation. The suppressor cell possesses the Ly 2, 3
antigens and not the Ly 1 antigen (Ly 1^-, 2^+, 3^+). As the
cytotoxic killer T cells, capable of killing cells from transplants
or tumors, are also Ly 1^-, 2^+, 3^+, there have been some suggestions that the *target* for the suppressor T cell is, in fact, the
helper T cell. On this idea, suppression would work by the
suppressor T cells killing the helper T cells. However, other experiments suggest that suppressor T cells work directly on B
cells, and the final word is not yet in on this issue. We shall discuss mechanisms of help and suppression much more fully in
Chapters 9 and 10.

So far we have seen that each of the major T cell subsets,
Ly 1^+, 2^-, 3^- and Ly 1^-, 2^+ 3^+, displays two sets of function,
the former helper functions and delayed hypersensitivity; the
latter suppressor functions and cytotoxic killing. It may be
necessary to break each subset into further sub-subsets. For
example, recent evidence shows that killer and suppressor cells
can be separated on the basis of yet another surface marker.

There is a third major subset of T lymphocytes which we have not mentioned yet, but which constitutes about half of the pool of T cells. These are lymphocytes possessing all of the antigens Ly 1, 2, and 3 (Ly 1^+, 2^+, 3^+ cells). The exact place of these cells in the scheme of things is not yet certain. These cells appear to be recent emigrants from the thymus and are rather short-lived. They may be a precursor type to the other two types, or they may possess some function yet to be discovered. Ly 1^+, 2^-, 3^- cells are several times more numerous than the Ly 1^-, 2^+, 3^+ in normal adult mice.

B Cell Subsets

The B lymphocytes are also not a homogeneous population. In fact, there are quite a number of cell surface markers which can be identified in some but not all B cells. Among those that are being assiduously studied are substances known as Fc receptors, C3 receptors, Ly 4 antigens, and Ia antigens. Furthermore, the Ig receptors on the B cell surface vary from cell to cell, some carrying IgM but no IgD, a few IgD but no IgM, while the majority display both classes. There is no point in going into too much detail about B cell subsets, however, because no consensus about a suitable classification has yet been reached; indeed we know little about why some B cells carry some markers but not others. As far as we know, the only function of B lymphocytes is to give rise to antibody-secreting cells, or alternatively to more B cells which can turn into antibody-forming cells should the antigen reenter the body sometime later. It is probable that B lymphocytes make up their minds, at some point in their maturation, about what class of antibody they will secrete when stimulated, but we need much more detailed knowledge about this. Similarly, it is a pity that we know so little about what makes some B cells produce beautiful and typical plasma cells on activation, while others may produce antibody-forming cells of rather nondescript morphological appearance, or even secretors that look virtually indistinguishable from normal small B lymphocytes. For the third edition of this book, we should have the data!

The Not-so-black Box

Niels K. Jerne, Director of the Basel Institute for Immunology and one of the most distinguished living immunologists, was once fond of classifying his research colleagues into three classes. The first group studies antigens—the nature and properties of chemical compounds that make them effective in various immunological situations. The second group studies antibodies— their chemistry, their physical properties, their size, shape, amino-acid sequence, and so forth. And then there is the third poor group (to which both he and I belong) which eschews the luxury of dealing with molecules that, however large or complex, possess a structure which must eventually be revealed by physical chemistry or biochemistry. Instead, these foolhardy individuals study the black box in between—the cells and organ systems which react to the antigens and make the antibodies. To most immunologists that black box seemed so impenetrable, so full of complexities, that the third group's task was considered hopelessly open-ended.

This categorization was moderately accurate a decade ago, but so spectacular has been the progress of the cellular immunologists that it has broken down almost completely. A substantial corpus of hard and respectable knowledge has accumulated about immunocytes. Increasingly, biochemists and molecular biologists who once would have classified cellular

immunology as too messy to warrant their attention are themselves delving into the fascinations of the lymphocyte, particularly of its cell membrane. The box is not so black after all, and
the dappled sunlight which has entered it will occupy most of
the rest of this book.

5

MOLECULAR STRATEGY OF IMMUNE RECOGNITION

Hოw can one know the unknown, recognize the unexpected? How can one react efficiently and precisely, when one has no prior warning of what, out of a myriad of potential stimuli, one will have to react against? These are the deep questions of immune recognition, an issue which Dr. Melvin Cohn has likened to only two others in physiology—the detoxification of poisons in the liver, and the learning processes of the brain. Two great humanists gave us the clue long before science addressed the question. Goethe said: "What one knows, one sees"; and Socrates believed that one could think constructively only about that which one already knew. The secret of the molecular strategy of immune recognition lies in the laying down of a preexistent large repertoire of recognition units, and then arranging for elements thereof to be called forth as occasions arise.

In the whole of its century-long history as an independent discipline, immunology has always bristled with vigorous con-

troversies. It is now rather fun to look into some of the literature of the late nineteenth century and to see the intense heat
and personal clashes which theories of immunology generated
even then. On occasion, the invective outshone the scientific
results in both scope and quality! In the present era of "Big Science" we tend to be less direct and more polite in our criticisms;
but wherever immunologists meet, animated discussions on how
cells *really do* make antibodies flourish well into the night. While
this very observation underscores the fact that we do not have a
full picture of the process, it will indicate where the cutting edge
of immunology is to be found. A commitment to achieving a
greater understanding of the mechanisms by which animals can
manufacture such a vast variety of different immunoglobulins
unites all workers in the field.

The first coherent theory of antibody formation was Ehrlich's
"side-chain" theory, published in 1897. The essence of this
formulation was that cells had chemical groupings or side-
chains, some of which, by pure chance, would fit to the chemical
groupings of the antigen. This naturally would interfere with
whatever was the normal function of the side-chain in the cell;
for this reason the cell would regenerate more side-chains to try
to compensate. Ehrlich claimed that "the antitoxins represent
nothing more than the side-chains reproduced in excess during
regeneration and are therefore pushed off from the protoplasm
—thus to exist in a free state." By modern standards, this theory
is too vague, but it does contain one vitally important notion
which has not only survived but has actually come to dominate
modern thinking. This is that cells can manufacture antibodies
before the antigen has come on the scene.

Karl Landsteiner's work put Ehrlich's thinking into temporary
eclipse. Landsteiner devoted himself to a most methodical analysis of the antibodies that can be synthesized against diverse small
chemical groupings or haptens. It soon became clear that the
recognition and discriminatory capacity of antibodies was immense. It did not seem plausible that any cell should willy-nilly

be synthesizing such a vast variety of "side chains." Rather, it was believed that the antigen induced some chemical change in the cell's synthetic machinery. This view gained general, if somewhat vague, acceptance. Professor Felix Haurowitz, lately of the University of Indiana, gave it cohesive existence when he formulated what has come to be known as the direct template theory of antibody formation. This straightforward chemical theory claimed that the antigen entered the antibody-forming cell and acted as a template or dye against which the globulin molecules folded themselves. Naturally, the globulin would assume a shape complementary to that of the antigen. It would, in fact, become a specific antibody.

A number of authors, and particularly Burnet, took issue with the direct template theory, chiefly on the grounds that it failed to explain many biological phenomena of immunity, including memory and tolerance. However, no really satisfactory alternative idea came forward until 1955. In that year, Jerne formulated his "natural selection theory" of antibody formation. At the time, it seemed quite unorthodox and a little outrageous. Jerne's own experimental work had dealt extensively with natural antibodies. These are antibodies present in the serum of animals that have had no known exposure to the antigen concerned. If one uses extremely sensitive methods for the detection of antibodies, it is not unusual to find that normal, healthy adult animals contain antibodies to all of a large variety of bacteria and viruses. Of course, the concentration of such antibodies in the serum is very low. Jerne argued that, had we methods of sufficient sensitivity, all conceivable antibodies might be present in the circulation. There are a total of over ten million trillion antibody molecules in the blood of a person. If one believes that immunoglobulins are synthesized into quite random patterns by lymphoid cells, this would present a vast number of potential locks, which surely could fit with any conceivable antigenic key. From this basic tenet, Jerne went on to postulate that any antigen injected into the body would soon meet with a corresponding natural antibody molecule. This complex would then be taken up by a phagocytic cell. From there on, the antigen would cease to play any useful role, but the antibody would serve as a template for its own reproduction. Thus the final end result would be a great acceleration of the rate of synthesis of that particular variant of natural antibody which fitted the recently injected antigen. The very greatly increased amount would now be readily detectable by conventional techniques and would give all the appearances of a specific new molecule. In fact, it would represent nothing more than the "iceberg," which had been present but submerged all this time, suddenly poking its tip above water.

In retrospect, it is easy to see how Jerne's theory bears many similarities to Ehrlich's original views, though it was conceived totally independently. It is now outmoded in a number of respects, but it certainly helped to restream modern thinking in immunology and accelerated the search for more precise knowledge.

Principles of Protein Production

We must here interrupt our historical analysis of theories of antibody formation and review a closely related but more general topic. The 1950s saw tremendous growth in our knowledge of the basic nature of protein production by cells in general, and in fact revealed that template theories suffered from grave defects. We have mentioned that DNA is a molecule made up of four bases (adenine, thymine, guanine, and cytosine) linked together by phosphate and sugar residues. The DNA of the cell contains its genetic code. The string of symbols coding for one protein is called a gene. It is believed that proteins are synthesized when a particular gene coding for that particular protein is activated or unlocked. The actual nature of this gene derepression, as it is termed, is complex. Frequently it involves the entry of some inducer molecule into the cell. When a gene is switched on, a coded copy of it is made in the form of messenger RNA. The ribosome, together with other nucleic acids and enzymes in the cell, does a good job of decoding. It makes a protein, the amino-acid sequence of which is inexorably determined by the sequence of triplets of bases in the gene. Therefore information in protein synthesis clearly flows from DNA to RNA to protein and not in the reverse direction. Proteins coming into the cell may change the rate of protein synthesis, lock or unlock genes, and perform all kinds of regulatory tasks. But one thing they cannot do is to alter the sequence of amino acids in a protein being synthesized. So, if an antigen did enter a cell and dictate to that cell the formation of an entirely new protein structure, it would be contravening all the known laws of protein synthesis.

There are, in fact, some exceptions to Crick's dogma of information flow. Some cancer-producing viruses possess an enzyme called reverse transcriptase which can make DNA copies of an RNA template, a stratagem which these RNA viruses may use to infiltrate themselves—or rather master plates of themselves—into the very genes of the infected cell. However, this is still a far cry from a protein conveying genetic information *not* for the formation of itself but rather for the formation of a complementary structure. Molecular biologists rejected direct template theories on theoretical grounds even before proof of selective theories came forward.

Clonal Selection Theory

In 1957, two leading immunologists came out independently with a theory which faced up to the above truths fully and which has now been formally proven as far as the B cell is concerned.

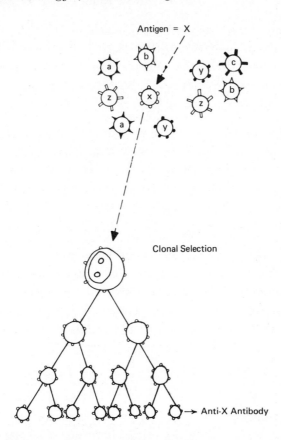

Figure 5–1. The clonal selection theory of antibody formation.

A simple view of this theory is presented in Figure 5–1. The two workers were Sir Macfarlane Burnet, my predecessor as Director of the Walter and Eliza Hall Institute of Medical Research, and Dr. David W. Talmage of the University of Colorado. They accepted the view that the information for the synthesis of all possible immunoglobulins must already be present in an unstimulated animal. They agreed further with Jerne that a base level of synthesis of all immunoglobulins was occurring. However, instead of envisaging a returning globulin molecule as the accelerator of synthesis, they placed the emphasis on replicating cells. This theory was termed the clonal selection theory. It predicted that lymphocytes came in a large variety of different patterns. Each lymphocyte was genetically fitted to synthesize one type of antibody. When an antigenic stimulus came, it had no effect on the bulk of lymphocytes, but selected for stimulation only those that were already making a corresponding antibody at a low rate. Such cells would have a sticky layer of the antibody on their surface, making a suitable receptor for the antigen or processed antigen. The result of stimulation of the selected cell would be the triggering of cell division in the previously resting cell, and the creation of a series of offspring. The name for such a series of progeny derived from a single ancestral cell is a clone—hence the name clonal selection. Two phenomena would be predicted from the theory: only a very small portion of all lymphocytes would respond to a given antigen; and one cell would always form only one antibody.

Impact of Knowledge of Immunoglobulin Structure on Theories of Antibody Diversity

The direct template theory, by which everything depended on how an antibody molecule folded itself during formation, was dealt a serious blow when it was realized that the final, coiled shape of a protein was wholly dependent on its amino-acid sequence. Indeed, proteins could be chemically unfolded into long strands, and when the chemical conditions causing this were reversed, they coiled right up again into their original, native shape. The coup de grace came experimentally when I, with the help of Dr. G. L. Ada, showed that an antibody-forming cell, with thousands of antibody factories in its cytoplasm, contained no detectable antigen inside it, even when we used techniques that would have spotted as few as four molecules. Independent of these considerations, knowledge was being gathered about immunoglobulin structure which proved that different antibodies had different amino-acid sequences and that the secret of antibody diversity was tied up in the V domains of immunoglobulin light and heavy chains, and in the genes coding for these. As the instructive theories of antibody formation were fading, however, the selective theories found themselves confronting new issues.

Formal Proof of Clonal Selection

As a thesis topic for my Ph.D. studies under Burnet, I was given the task of gathering some evidence for or against the new clonal selection theory. It seemed to me that a first approach might be to inject an animal with two or three different antigens and to ask whether a given, single antibody-forming cell would always make only one antibody against one antigen, as clonal selection would predict, or whether it would sometimes make two or three specificities, as the animal as a whole was doing. The trouble was that experiments on the cellular basis of antibody formation had, until that time, been done not with one cell but with tens of millions of cells. With the help of Dr. Joshua Lederberg I solved the technical problems of isolating and measuring the antibody secreted by single cells. This involved much tedious micromanipulation, though watching the efforts of a single cell's antibody to paralyze the flippers of a single, swimming bacterium was also great fun! The results were clear-cut: one cell always made one antibody.

This observation, however, was only a first step. It could well have been that a B lymphocyte had receptors for many antigens, but that the first antigen hitting a cell committed it to the formation of only that antibody, in much the same way that one female egg cell is inherently capable of being fertilized by any one of the myriad sperms, but, once fertilized by one, firmly rejects all others. Fortunately, the topic soon became a popular research question, and many laboratories have contributed to its solution. First it was shown that B lymphocytes do have receptors for antigens on their surface, namely immunoglobulin molecules. Then it turned out that B cells were heterogeneous in their capacity to react with antigens. When a large number of cells was taken from the spleen of an unimmunized normal adult animal, and mixed with a protein antigen that had been tagged with a radioactive marker, only a small proportion (say, one in 5000) of the cells absorbed enough antigen onto their surface to suggest immunologically specific binding. Furthermore, if such antigen-binding B cells were removed from the lymphocyte suspension, or were rendered impotent by plastering highly radioactive antigen onto their surface, damaging the DNA of the cells, then that lymphocyte population lost the capacity to form antibodies to that particular antigen while retaining reactivity against other unrelated antigens. All of this was consistent with clonal selection, but not formal proof.

What was required was to isolate from the vast and heterogeneous multitude of normal B lymphocytes one cell, with receptors for a specific, preferably very simple, antigen. Then that single cell should be taken, stimulated with the given antigen, and should unfailingly make a clone of progeny cells, all forming the corresponding antibody. Stimulated with other antigens, the cell should fail to respond. The pathway to that experiment was tortuous and fraught with ghastly technical problems, but in 1976, after nearly 20 years of struggle, my colleagues and I finally reached it. With Dr. Werner Haas and Miss Beverley Pike, I was able to fractionate a subset of lymphocytes with receptors for a given hapten termed NIP, and to culture these lymphocytes in plastic containers in an incubator, stimulating them with the NIP hapten hooked onto a carrier protein. The cells, incapable of synthesizing an antibody to another hapten DNP, initiated the formation of an antibody-producing clone—not one time in 10,000, as the unfractionated population had done, but one time in three and a half. Bearing in mind that many lymphocytes die in tissue culture, for various uninteresting technical reasons, we can conclude that this experiment comes fairly close to providing formal proof of the clonal selection theory.

We are farther away in our attempts to prove the uniqueness of the antigen-combining specificity of the receptors on a given single T lymphocyte. Suffice it to say that all the indications suggest that clonal selection operates among T cells as well.

How is the finding of one lymphocyte/one receptor specificity to be reconciled with the observation that one B lymphocyte frequently has two different classes of immunoglobulin on it, IgM and IgD? This is no problem. In those cases, the light chain (be it κ or λ) is identical in the two classes, and the heavy chain V domain is also identical. Thus, every single Ig molecule on that cell displays exactly the same antibody-combining site, made up of one V_L and one V_H domain. All that differs is that some of the receptors have one kind of handle, others another. This in no way affects the antigen-combining specificity of the receptor molecules.

Generating the Immunological Repertoire

It is indeed difficult to accept intuitively that a repertoire of antibody types adequate to cope with any conceivable invader preexists in the animal. However, a man has a trillion lymphocytes and, even given that it is likely that not all of these differ in receptor pattern, this still leaves a lot of possibilities for diversity. An important fact to bear in mind is that the antibody system is *degenerate* and *redundant*. There are more ways than one of making a combining site for a given antigenic determinant (let alone a whole antigen molecule), and one given combining site can serve as an antibody for different antigenic determinants. The exquisite specificity of *antisera* which Landsteiner observed was at least in part a property of *populations* of diverse antibody molecules. Thus, a mosaic of antigenic determinants can be discriminated with exquisite specificity from a second mosaic through the combined specificities of the two sets of antibody molecules in the two antisera.

It has been estimated that the number of different kinds of antibodies capable of being made by an adult mouse is around 10 million, a reasonable estimate considering that a mouse possesses some thousand million lymphocytes in all, of which half are T cells. How does the body generate the repertoire of 10^7 different kinds of watchful B cells that stand in readiness to produce their particular antibody (or *clonotype*)? Whatever the mechanism may be, it is very specialized and of the utmost interest to geneticists and embryologists as well as immunologists.

At one extreme of theorizing, we have the strict germ line theory. This states that for every different V domain of Ig chains there exists a specific gene in the DNA of the fertilized egg, just as there exist genes for the synthesis of hemoglobin, insulin, and all the myriad proteins which that animal must make. Then, by a process which is essentially only an example of cellular differentiation, and the assumption of specialized gene expression that we see in so many cells (after all, pancreas cells don't think and brain cells don't make insulin!), the different lymphocytes come to express different V gene products—one V gene for the light chain and one for the heavy. The theory obviously requires the presence within each cell of a large, tandem array of V genes, one for each possible V domain. This would occupy a great slab of the DNA which the cell has for its coding functions. Nevertheless, the number need not be so large as to be ridiculous. Suppose that there were $10^{3.5}$ (or about 3200) V_H genes and $10^{3.5}$ V_L genes in each cell, as each V_H region could pair with each V_L region, this would make $10^{3.5} \times 10^{3.5}$ different $V_H V_L$ pairs—in other words 10^7 antibody sites. The theory leaves open a number of questions, including the mechanism whereby nature ensures that, with all of this genetic potential locked inside it, each cell expresses only one $V_L V_H$ pair. Existing evidence (and it is not final) from direct studies of lymphocyte nucleic acids makes it seem unlikely that there are so many V gene copies in the germ line.

At the other extreme, there is the original somatic mutation theory of Burnet. This requires that there be only one gene for the V region of each of the Ig chains. However, a special genetic process confers a high rate of mutation on these genes as the pre-B cells and B cells divide in the body. The result is that the limited amount of information in the germ line is diversified into a large repertoire during the actual lifetime of the animal. The non-germ cells (or somatic cells) of the body itself have to perform the task of diversification, not the traditional Darwinian processes of evolution. Thus antibody formation is a kind of natural selection in the microcosm of the body's own tissues.

In its extreme form, this theory cannot be correct, as the different subgroups (see Chapter 3) of the V domains could not have arisen from a single V gene that had mutated several times during one life span. They are simply too different from each other. There must be one V gene per V domain subgroup. The trouble is, no one can say for sure how many subgroups there really are for V_κ, V_λ and V_H, the three genes we are concerned with. In the mouse, where lambda light chains are surprisingly sparse, making up only three percent of all light chains, there appears to be only one V_λ subgroup, but this is clearly an exceptional situation. One reasonable estimate puts the number of V_L and V_H subgroups (and thus the number of tandemly arrayed V_L and V_H genes) at 30 to 100 each. If this is correct, there would be enough information in the germ line to make 30×30 to 100×100 antibody sites, or 900 to 10,000 sites. Then, only a much more modest (though still substantial) rate of somatic mutation would be required to generate a full repertoire of 10^7 (or more) antibody types. This theory has many adherents at the time of writing.

Other views are possible, such as mechanisms for arranging high rates of DNA breakage and incorrect repair in those sections of the V region genes that code for the hypervariable regions (see Chapter 3); or mechanisms which insert virus-like particles (episomes) into these same regions. Obviously only deeper study of lymphocyte DNA itself will solve the problem.

Translocation of V and C Genes

One final fascinating genetic sidelight of immunological theory must be mentioned. Proteins are made to the dictates of a messenger RNA and a messenger RNA is a transcribed copy of a single gene. All the evidence indicates that the messenger RNA of an antibody chain is not especially different from any other messenger RNA. It is a single thread of code units. Yet, it is a transcribed copy of *two different* genes, the V gene and the C gene. There are many V genes (just how many we don't know) but only one C gene for each class of chain. Moreover, a single V gene, inside a single cell, can come into contact with two different C genes. Thus, in a cell possessing IgM and IgD receptors, with identical combining sites, a given V_H gene appears to make contact simultaneously with the C genes for μ and δ heavy chains. We presume a process of *gene translocation* must take place by some kind of cutting of the DNA strand followed by appropriate splicing. This alone is not enough because it must happen twice over; each V gene must be present as two repeats in the DNA strand (which is perfectly possible) or else must be duplicated before translocation to the two C genes.

All of these mechanisms involve unique postulates, revolutionary in their implications for molecular biology and genetics. No doubt our ideas will seem as primitive to twenty-first-century immunologists as Ehrlich's and Landsteiner's do today. I, for one, hope so, because as soon as a field of science stops changing, it becomes a dull, dead thing. The main value of the various theories over the decades has been to crystallize existing data into a self-consistent picture and to catalyze creative experimentation. If they can continue to do this, it does not matter much how rapidly they succeed each other!

6

EVOLUTION OF
THE IMMUNE SYSTEM

Over a thousand million years ago the first signs of life appeared on earth, almost certainly in the sea. The fundamental unit of living matter is the cell, a tiny globule consisting of a nucleus, some surrounding protoplasm, termed *cytoplasm*, and bounded by a cell membrane. Many of the earliest living species consisted of only one cell—the so-called unicellular organisms. The most successful of these tiny creatures survive to the present day and include the well-known amoebas and also important parasites such as the malarial plasmodia. However, from the very beginning, life was a competitive affair. As the primitive species multiplied, food became scarce. When a cell divided, sometimes the daughter cell was not an exact replica. Usually the copying error resulted in a defect of some sort, but occasionally, by sheer chance, the progeny was more fitted to the competitive environment. Nature seized upon this apparently haphazard method to evolve the different species. Over the millennia a vast variety of different forms of life were generated.

A great leap forward came when cells grouped together to form multicellular organisms. Slowly, more and more complex animals and plants arose.

Phagocytosis

Almost from the beginning, species needed ways of defending themselves in order to preserve their integrity. The most primitive of defense mechanisms is possessed even by the lowly amoeba. It is a combined mechanism of defense and nutrition, based on the principle: "If I don't eat it, it might eat me." The process is known as *phagocytosis*. The electron microscope has given us an accurate picture of the sequence of events involved, and this is shown in Figure 6–1. Let us suppose a particle such as a bacterium approaches our amoeba. Contact is made, and soon the cell membrane of the amoeba becomes indented. The particle is dragged further into the cell and becomes progressively surrounded by membrane turned outside-in. As ingestion is completed, the neck of the long invagination fuses. The bacterium thus finds itself surrounded on all sides by inverted cell membrane. It is inside a little pouch, which we term a *vacuole*. Now the process of destruction of the cannibalized prisoner can begin. The cell contains a number of powerful substances, termed *digestive enzymes*, which can help to eat away the macromolecules making up the bacterium by breaking them down into their component building blocks. In order that these enzymes do not destroy the cell they are meant to serve, they too live in little pouches, termed *lysosomes*. Now it is simply a question of several of the enzyme-containing lysosomes meeting and fusing with the vacuole containing the bacterium. The digestive enzymes are thus jetted into the enlarged phagocytic vacuole or "phagolysosome" without ever once having endangered the living cytoplasm of the cell. They break the bacterium

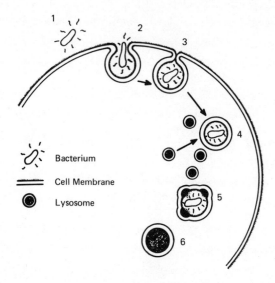

Figure 6–1.   Schematic view of phagocytosis. 1: A bacterium close to the cell surface. 2: Entering commences
through invagination of the cell membrane. 3: The invagination is about to separate from the cell membrane.
4: Lysosomes approach the vacuole. 5: Lysosomes fuse
with the vacuole and discharge their enzymes. 6: Digestion
of bacterium nearly completed.

down progressively until it disappears altogether. The now
innocuous and broken building blocks can be used by the
amoeba for its own nutrition and growth.

    One of the key advantages of the multicellular organisms over
their unicellular ancestors is that not every cell has to do every
job. The advantages of specialization were not discovered in our
century, even though the concept has been developed to an
unprecedented extent in our society! As evolution progressed,
certain parts of an animal or plant took over certain tasks, and
complex organ systems gradually developed. In this way, the
task of phagocytosis, rather than being the duty of every cell,

was delegated to certain specialized cells which, not unnaturally, we call *phagocytes*.

Here we must pause to pay tribute to the great Russian zoologist, Elie Metchnikoff, whose work provided the basis of most of our current knowledge about these vital scavenger cells, and whose pioneering studies received the Nobel Prize for medicine in 1908. Metchnikoff found that species as primitive as the larvae of starfish, which do not possess circulatory or nervous systems, had a whole army of mobile cells to help them get rid of foreign matter. He was the first to show that the result of an infection could depend on the efficiency of these little guardians of health. In fact, Metchnikoff found himself the center of a heated scientific controversy which involved many biologists at the turn of the century. Which was the more important in immunity, antibody or scavenger cells? Now we know the truth of the matter: both are important, and a collaboration between antibodies and cells provides a defense mechanism more efficient than either alone.

The type of analysis we have just described is the fruit of research involving a creative interplay of microscopy and electron microscopy to gain information about the structure of tissues and cells; biophysics necessary for the separation of bits of cells from one another prior to analysis; and biochemistry to determine what is the chemical task of each separated bit. The value of this overall approach was recognized in 1974 by the award of the Nobel Prize to three pioneers. Among the trio was Dr. Christian de Duve, the discoverer of the lysosome.

Emergence of Specific Immunity

Phagocytosis, as we have seen, is a very primitive phenomenon. Antibodies are made only by animals much higher on the evolutionary scale than the larvae of the starfish. In fact, for many millions of years, phagocytosis seems to have been the standby. A complex array of nonspecific barriers against the outside world was developed over this period. These included not only the obvious mechanical barriers such as skin, scales, or shells, but also a variety of secretions and enzymes. One good example is the important substance that Sir Alexander Fleming identified some years before his even greater discovery of penicillin. This is lysozyme, a digestive ferment capable of killing many bacteria, and present in high concentration in quite diverse biological fluids such as egg white and tears. These substances are nonspecific in that they do not constitute a tailor-made response to a particular invasion, in contrast to the antibody response. Rather, these nonspecific factors represent a general background of defense which appeared to do a good job until nature "turned up" the more sophisticated specific immune response.

Scientists have spent many long hours searching for antibodies in nonvertebrate species. Every now and then an isolated report appears in the technical literature concerning the possibility of antibody formation in sea anemones, horseshoe crabs, or some other lowly form of life. However, so far none of these studies has yielded really convincing evidence of the existence of an antibody defense mechanism similar to that in mammals. As we shall see, it is important that the search for some primordial type of antibody should go on. It could provide a vital missing link in our knowledge of the evolution of the immune system.

The first indication of the appearance of a specific, new type of defense mechanism has been traced back some 480 million years ago. At that time, marine species developed a primitive type of backbone. It was, as yet, made only of cartilage. The more sturdy vertebral column, consisting largely of bones, came later. The oldest type of cartilaginous fish, or cyclostome, is fortunately known to us not only through fossil remains. Two examples have survived to the present day. The two major groups are the hagfish (*Eptatrediae*) and the lampreys (*Petromyzodinae*). Hagfish are found only in salt water, lampreys in both fresh and salt water. By catching these primitive fish and keeping them for some weeks or months in a suitable marine laboratory, one can do direct experiments to test their primitive defense system and to see whether they are capable of forming antibodies. These species possess a primitive type of blood lymphocyte and can make an IgM-like antibody response of rather poor avidity. Cell-mediated immunity is also present, as is a rudimentary thymus.

In higher fish the immune process is much more efficient. For example, in the elasmobranchs, such as the sharks, the thymus is well developed and there are large numbers of lymphocytes in the spleen. In the same organ we can identify a new type of cell, especially powerful in antibody production, the plasma cell. Thus, when we look in the serum of a shark some days after the injection of an antigen, we find a much higher concentration of antibodies than we would have found in a lamprey. All of these antibodies are IgM in nature. Chemical analysis shows that the IgM is composed of heavy and light chains, as is the IgM of humans. Unlike the higher vertebrates, however, IgG has not yet made its appearance. For some reason, the bigger and apparently more complex molecule arose first, and the smaller, highly avid immunoglobulin type was evolved later.

Fish can also reject grafts briskly, displaying the cellular arm of the immune response. In fact, surgery in goldfish can be quite good fun! It is simply a question of pulling out a scale and neatly substituting one from a different fish, preferably of a slightly different color. Such grafts heal very well. However, within some days the immune machinery sends the relentless lymphocyte policemen to the area and the graft is promptly rejected.

From fish we can learn another basic bit of biology. Most chemical reactions in the body—that is, *biochemical* reactions—go on most efficiently at around 37° C, which represents blood heat for warm-blooded creatures like ourselves. Fish, however, are cold-blooded. In general they assume the body temperature of the water around them. Their blood heats up and cools down as the water in which they swim becomes warmer or colder—it very rarely gets as warm as 37° C. When we study either graft rejection or antibody formation in fish, we can quickly discover that they reject grafts faster and form antibodies more quickly and in higher concentration when the water is kept relatively warm rather than cool. Of course, the range of variation in man's blood temperature is much less. Even in a serious infection it rarely gets above 41° C. To my knowledge, no one has made a detailed study of how such high temperatures affect rates of antibody formation. It would be interesting if a high fever in fact slightly accelerated the process in a child sick with an infection.

Anyone who has ever had a boil or a carbuncle does not need to be reminded what a lymph node is. It is the lump in the arm-pit or groin which swells up and becomes sore when the bacteria (or antigens from them) reach it. The lymph nodes are impor-tant sites of antibody production. Fish do not possess lymph nodes. These structures first appeared in a very restricted way in the amphibians—the animals that learned to crawl out of the sea and to live both on land and under water. Frogs and toads are typical examples of modern amphibians that are easily ob-tained and conveniently studied in the laboratory. In The Walter and Eliza Hall Institute, we have done quite a bit of work with toads. When placed in wet sawdust they live quite happily, be-come terribly lazy, and appear to eat practically nothing. Yet they form antibodies at a great rate, in fact practically as well as rats and mice. The amphibians make both IgM and IgG.

In one respect, however, their immune system is not fully evolved. This is in the degree to which they exhibit immunologi-cal memory. One of the hallmarks of a mammalian immune response is that a second shot of antigen, given two weeks or more after the first shot, elicits a "booster" response; this is a rapid burst of antibody formation more intense than that which followed the first injection. This quality of remembering the lessons of the first reaction is termed *immunological memory*.

Amphibians have a weak memory system and are much inferior to human beings in at least this regard! Of course, immunological memory has nothing to do with the memory function of the brain. The cellular basis of immunological memory will be discussed in Chapter 11.

The next and last major step forward in the evolution of the immune system took place in the primitive mammals themselves. Unfortunately we do not have any ideally suitable mammals which are directly representative of the chain linking reptiles to modern mammals. However, in Australia, there are two examples of very ancient mammals that are much closer to the common ancestors of all present-day mammals than are the mice, rabbits, and guinea pigs which have been so extensively studied. These quaint Australian natives are the egg-laying mammals or *monotremes*. Two varieties can be found in their bush habitat: the echidna or spiny anteater, and the platypus. In their appearance and bodily functions they exhibit some features that are bird-like, some that are fish-like, and some that are mammalian. Study of the lymph system of these species has shown that they possess a very large number of quite tiny lymph nodes. Microscopic examination shows the presence of special little knots of rapidly dividing lymphocytes which we term *germinal centers*. We believe these to have an important function in immunological memory. As you may have guessed, study of the antibody response of echidnas shows, for the first time in evolution, the existence of a really sturdy antibody memory system.

Thus we can see that the highly efficient immunological apparatus that modern mammals like human beings possess passed through a large number of different stages, many of which we can trace through detailed examination of lower species. The brief outline that has been given is an example of an important branch of modern science, namely, comparative physiology. Nature always designs things cunningly. If we look only at the most advanced products of her ingenuity, such as the human brain, the hormonal control system, or the immune defense mechanism, we may become bewildered by the complexities which confront us. A patient, historical search backwards through evolution can often simplify and illuminate the problem.

Molecular Evolution of Antibodies

Our thinking about the variable and constant halves of the immunoglobulin light chain was helped by a look at a few words written in English rather than in the symbolism of amino acids and proteins. Therefore, let us look at two more words:

EPILEPSY
MATHEMATIC

What do these words have in common? Simply this: there is homology between the two halves of each word. Epilepsy consists of eight letters; and two letters in positions 1 and 2 are repeated in positions 5 and 6. There is even more homology between the two halves of mathematic. Here 1, 2, and 3 each correspond with 6, 7, and 8.

One of the most interesting findings that has come out of an analysis of amino-acid sequence of immunoglobulin chains is that there are readily definable homologies between the two halves of the light chain, between portions of the heavy and the light chains, and between light chains of different animal species. For example, the last four amino acids of mouse light chains are asparagine-arginine-asparagine-cystine. The last four of human light chains are asparagine-arginine-glycine-cystine. The homology is striking: three of the four are identical. Other similar stretches can be found, although the homology is usually not quite so close.

This has allowed the speculation to emerge that *all* antibodies evolved from some ancestral protein. The domain hypothesis of immunoglobulin structure discussed in Chapter 3, which has been strongly supported by recent X-ray crystallographic evidence, is also consistent with the idea that *gene duplication* is at the root of the evolution of the immune system. Suppose there were some primordial gene coding, for example, for a cell surface molecule of about 110 amino acids (the size of one immunoglobulin domain). Suppose it duplicated several times, and the members of the resulting tandem series each underwent their own processes of mutation and selection. Sooner or later (like the famous monkeys bashing away steadily at their typewriters) a set of molecules sufficiently variant from each other as to constitute a repertoire of recognition units could emerge. If it turned out that possession of a large repertoire conferred survival advantages on individuals possessing it, evolution would certainly "encourage" the process to continue. The array of germ line V and C genes could have arisen like this. Duplication of V genes would gradually have enlarged the recognition repertoire, duplication of C genes the number of biologically different classes of antibodies, subserving different physiological roles.

These exciting speculations can be taken even further. It has recently been discovered that a molecule about the size of one Ig domain, 12,000 molecular weight, and strongly homologous to the C domains of IgG, exists on the surface of every cell. It functions as the light chain of a set of molecules, known as *histocompatibility antigens*. These molecules, which we shall encounter again several times, are important in graft rejection and also in cellular interactions. Could it be that preglobulin molecules have some universally important role, say in embryological differentiation, or some aspect of maintenance of tissue integrity? Once again, we find immunologists milling hard around some of the central questions in biology. Experimentally, it may still turn out that scientists looking for molecules on the surface of the macrophages of Metchnikoff's starfish larvae will provide clues of general fascination.

7

ANATOMY FOR IMMUNE BATTLES

EVEN a superficial knowledge of military strategy allows us to see the advantages of a national defense system that is diversified and deployed. Most countries have not only an army but a navy and air force as well. Moreover, troops are not concentrated in just a single area, nor are individual soldiers scattered randomly and singly over a whole country. Rather, there are organized units stationed at critical, carefully chosen, and separated key points. If we take a somewhat deeper look at the defense establishment, two of many factors we must consider are where the new recruits come from, and how they are to be trained efficiently. Similarly, when we think about bodily defense, we must consider not only the different types of cells and the location and nature of the organs in which they are concentrated. We must also give some thought, in this chapter and the next, to the questions of the ultimate source and origin of these cells, and of any specialized "training" they may have to receive to fulfill their important task.

The Circulating Defenders

Before looking closely at lymph nodes, spleen, and other sites of antibody formation, let us start with a consideration of the cells floating in the bloodstream. A normal adult male will have about 10 pints of blood in his body: 45 percent of it is composed of cells, both red and white; 55 percent is composed of blood fluid which we term *plasma*. Fresh blood clots, and when the cells and proteinaceous material constituting the solid part of the clot are removed, a straw-colored fluid remains which we term *serum*. Serum is really the same as plasma but lacks the special clotting protein, *fibrinogen*. For a number of technical reasons immunologists tend to use serum rather than plasma when doing antibody studies, and they can express the antibody concentration as so many micrograms or milligrams of antibody per milliliter of serum.

The number of red cells in the blood staggers the imagination. There are about 5 billion per milliliter or 25 trillion in a whole adult. Red cells transport oxygen and have nothing to do with defense as such. White cells are much in the minority in the bloodstream—there is about one white cell for every 1,000 red cells. This still gives 5–10 million per milliliter. The white cells are considerably bigger than the red cells. If a thin test tube full of blood has a tiny quantity of an anti-clotting agent added to it and is allowed to stand, the red cells will settle to the bottom, the white cells will settle on top of them, and the plasma over the white cells. The little collar of white cells is perhaps one-hundredth rather than one-thousandth the height of the column of red cells. This is because the red cells are really flattened disks whereas the white cells are plump spheres of a slightly greater diameter and considerably greater volume. This collar of white cells actually looks white or whitish-yellow to the naked eye, hence the name. The technical name for the little collar of pure white cells is "buffy coat."

POLYMORPHONUCLEAR LEUCOCYTES

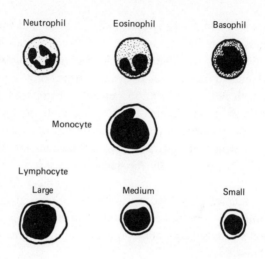

Figure 7–1. The main types of white blood cells.

In Figure 7–1, we can see the three major types of white blood cells, all of which have important and different defense functions. The most numerous cells are the polymorphonuclear leucocytes. This awkward name simply means "white cells with nuclei of many shapes" and refers to the fact that the nuclei of these cells are segmented and convoluted. A synonym for this class of cells is granulocyte, or simply "cell with granules," which illustrates another feature, namely, the presence in the cytoplasm of many round inclusions which resemble in some respects the lysosomes (already discussed and illustrated in Figure 6–1). This should provide a clue as to the prime function of granulocytes: they are highly efficient phagocytes. When bacteria enter the body, this category of cells represents a first line of attack. Within minutes, they march to the site of infection in large numbers and begin to engulf the invaders. (As we shall see, antibody production is slower to get going.)

There are three types of granulocytes, and the names given to them are derived from the way in which the cells take certain dyes. "Neutrophil" polymorphonuclear leucocytes like acidic and basic dyes equally; "eosinophils" stain selectively with acidic dyes such as eosin, a red dye; and "basophils" take up basic dyes, many of which are colored blue to purple. Blood specialists, whom we term hematologists, have devised mixtures of dyes which can stain the various types of granulocytes within minutes. Neutrophils are present in the largest number. They represent the standard model of polymorph, and when an infection of any degree of seriousness strikes, their frequency in the bloodstream can increase by a factor of five or more. Similarly, when their level in the blood is reduced, as it is in some diseases, a grave situation is created as it leaves the person unduly prone to infections of all sorts. Eosinophils are especially prominent in infections with parasites, such as various worms, and also in allergies. Basophils contain granules which rupture readily and release a variety of materials which increase inflammation. Most people think of the redness, heat, and swelling around infections as something bad. In fact, this complex process of inflammation is the body's way of bringing special help—more blood and more cells—to a danger area. The polymorphs in general play a key role in inflammation.

The factory for granulocytes is in the bone marrow and, to a much less important extent, in the spleen. Thus these cells are formed in the same organs as the red cells. Frequently, when the bone marrow is afflicted by disease, production of both red cells and white cells is depressed, and the number of each in the blood drops. The result can be expressed as "anemia" when there are too few red cells and "leucopenia" when there are too few white cells.

The second type of cell in the blood is the monocyte. The name is really an abbreviation of mononuclear leucocyte. These cells form only a small percent of the total number of cells, and represent another variant of phagocytic cell. This mobile blood pool of relatively young phagocytic cells readily enters the tissues and develops there into a larger and more active phagocyte called a "macrophage." In contrast to polymorphs which live for a few days only, macrophages can live for weeks or months. Macrophages are particularly common in liver, spleen, and lymph nodes, but are widely distributed throughout the whole body. The macrophage, which is really only a later developmental stage of the monocyte, does not itself form antibodies but plays a catalytic role in antibody formation. This will be discussed in Chapter 9.

The third type of cell in the blood is the most important from our point of view. It is the lymphocyte. Blood lymphocytes come in a wide range of sizes. When their diameters are measured under the microscope, they vary from 5 thousandths of a millimeter (5 microns, or simply 5 μ) to 15 μ. The larger the cell, the younger it is. Medium-sized lymphocytes are the progeny of large lymphocytes, small lymphocytes of medium-sized ones. The small lymphocytes can be remarkably long-lived. A goodly proportion circulate for months and even years. We have already noted that this simple classification by size does not tell us whether a lymphocyte is a T or B cell, what hierarchy it is in, or what subset.

The Third Circulation—Lymph and Lymphatics

The blood leaves the main left chamber of the heart by a big artery termed the *aorta*. Smaller branches are given off, which in turn have smaller branches, and finally end in tiny, thin-walled blood vessels termed *capillaries*. The vast network of capillaries permeates every organ and tissue of the body. It is this capillary bed which actually feeds oxygen and fuel to the cells composing the organs. The blood in the capillaries enters now progressively larger and larger vessels, the veins, which return to the right side of the heart. Now a second circulation sends blood to the lungs. Here the *arterial* blood is poor in oxygen; the capillaries trap oxygen from the air in the lungs, and the venous blood returns rich in oxygen to the left side of the heart.

During each circulation some fluid leaves the capillary bed and enters the tissue spaces. Why do the tissues not get water-logged? Because there exists a third circulation, one that is vital to our understanding of the immune response. The tissues them-selves are drained, not only by veins, but by a delicate system of thin-walled vessels called lymphatics. At their origins in the tissues, these vessels are open-ended and communicate with the spaces between cells. The tiniest lymphatics soon join to form larger lymphatics, and finally all end in large lymph vessels which empty into large veins. The fluid draining from the tissues is known simply as "lymph." Lymph mixes with the venous blood, and, just like it, circulates around again. As you can imagine, if the main lymph vessels draining, say, an arm or a leg *do* get blocked, considerable waterlogging will result. The leg will become swollen and soggy. This actually happens in the disease called elephantiasis, where parasitic worms lodge in the lymph vessels.

Lymph Nodes

Studded along the course of the lymphatics are a number of complicated filters, the lymph nodes. A schematic view of a lymph node is given in Figure 7–2. Before entering a lymph

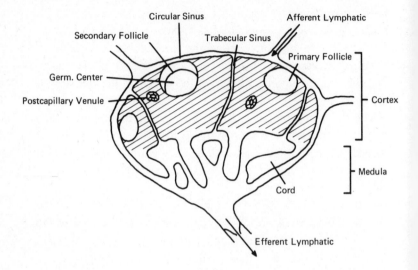

Figure 7–2. Schematic diagram of a section through a lymph node.

node, the lymphatic vessel breaks up into a number of small branches which are called "afferent" lymphatics, or lymphatics bringing lymph to the node. This distinguishes them from the vessel which leaves the node—the "efferent" lymphatic.

Have you ever had a badly poisoned toe? If so, you will know that the lymph nodes form a chain. The first area in which you notice a swollen gland is behind the knee, in a node that we call the *popliteal node*. Then you may notice the glands in the groin, or inguinal glands, enlarging. In other words, the efferent lymphatic vessel from the popliteal node becomes the *afferent* vessel for the inguinal node. The efferent vessel from the inguinal node will become the afferent for the next highest lymph node and so on until the lymph is discharged into the venous circulation. This whole series of elaborate filters has the twin jobs of removing foreign matter by phagocytosis and being a major site for antibody production and development of cell-mediated immunity.

Preparation of a Lymph Node Section

Before we take a closer look at Figure 7–2, which represents a section cut right through the middle of a lymph node, let us find out how knowledge of the cellular organization of tissues in general can be obtained. Nineteenth-century anatomists perfected a very ingenious method of preparing tissue sections which retain the chief cellular features of the living organ. We still use these techniques, though some improvements have been made. First, the lymph node, or any other organ, is placed in a hardening fluid or "fixative," which instantly kills the cells and precipitates the proteins and other macromolecules, thus preserving them in their correct relationship to each other. The best-known fixative is formalin. Alcohol, chloroform, and acetic acid are other examples of fixatives. Frequently, the best fixation is obtained by using mixtures of a number of fixatives.

When fixation is completed, after several hours or days, depending on the tissue, the next step is to remove all water from the preparation. This is usually done by soaking the specimen in alcohol solutions of increasing concentration, for example, 70, 90, and 95 percent, and absolute alcohol. Several changes of solution at each strength are usually used. Next, the alcohol is cleared away by a solvent such as xylol or chloroform, and then the whole tissue is impregnated with paraffin wax by placing it in an oven in a series of solutions of hot paraffin. The paraffin is then cooled, and it sets hard both within and around the organ. Then it is trimmed into a nice, square block which can be mounted on a slicing machine, or *microtome*. This machine cuts slices or "sections" of 5μ to 10μ thickness (1cm = 10mm = 10,000 μ). This is about the thickness of a single cell. Now one must remove the paraffin, fill the tissue with water again, and stain the rehydrated section with a variety of dyes.

This sounds like a very complex procedure, and one may well wonder whether it is worth all the trouble. In fact, an enormous proportion of the knowledge about the structure and function of the body has come from application of this procedure. As regards normal tissues, the study of stained sections forms a part of anatomy; the name of this branch of science is. *histology.* When it comes to diseases, knowledge of how cells go wrong is obtained from sections of the diseased organs; this branch of medicine is termed *pathology.* Frequently a surgeon plans his whole line of attack on information given to the pathologist by a section of some lump or other abnormality. Clearly histology, pathology, and sections in general are vital to both biology and medicine.

The microscope uses light as an energy source, and a variety of lens systems give us magnifications of up to 1,000 or slightly more. Beyond this, the light microscope cannot go. However, if electrons are used as the energy source and electromagnetic fields are made to act as lenses, a microscope with a magnifying power of 100,000 can be built. This we term the electron microscope. While the technique of preparing sections for the electron microscope differs in some important details, the principles are as outlined above. The sections are about 100 times thinner than in light microscopy. So far electron microscopy has been used mainly as a research tool, but it is creeping into the field of diagnostic pathology.

The Cortex and Medulla of Lymph Nodes

With this preamble we can turn again to Figure 7–2. The afferent lymphatics enter a thin, fluid-filled space which coats the
whole of the roughly spherical node. This space is called the
circular lymph sinus. The node under this can be thought of as a
shell and a core. The outer shell is termed the *cortex*, the core
is the *medulla*. Most of the fluid entering the circular sinus
travels straight to the medulla by thin channels termed *trabecu-
lar sinuses*. A significant minority of the fluid, however, passes
into the cortex by small pores in the outer lining of the circular
sinus.

The cortex of the node is made up mainly of lymphocytes,
the medulla of phagocytic cells, chiefly macrophages, and of
antibody-forming plasma cells. Both areas, however, are quite
complex and variegated. The cortex contains two aspects that
we will meet again: (1) special, rounded and densely packed
collections of lymphocytes and antigen-trapping cells, called
lymphoid follicles; and (2) veins with unusually thick walls and
a strange function, called postcapillary venules. The medulla is
made up of two parts: (1) cords, which stick into the medulla
from the cortex like many fingers poking into a partially filled
balloon; and (2) open spaces, or sinuses, where many macrophages lie in wait to capture foreign material present in the
lymph. The whole lymph node is a dynamic area. Cells enter
and leave; sinuses fill and empty; the node gets big when antigens
hit it, and subsequently shrinks again. The cords are perhaps the
most prone to change. When all is quiet, they are narrow and
inconspicuous. When infections come, they balloon out and fill
up with plasma cells, becoming the most prominent portion of
the medulla.

In Chapter 6 we mentioned an entity termed the *germinal
center*. We can now place this in its correct setting. The lymph-

oid follicles of the cortex are quite small before any antigens strike the node. When they are stimulated, however, they become much larger and a central core of large, rapidly dividing lymphocytes can be seen. The little, inconspicuous, unstimulated follicles are termed *primary follicles*. The follicles which develop after antigenic stimulation and contain germinal centers are called *secondary follicles*.

While both T and B cells move in and out of lymph nodes, and also within them, each class of cell has its favorite niche or living area within the node. The primary and secondary follicles consist largely of B cells. The medullary cords, with their rich content of plasma cells (which are activated B cells), are another B area. With the exception of a small rim of cells just beneath the circular sinus, and particularly the deeper areas of the cortex, the diffuse cortical tissue contains mainly T cells. If a strong cell-mediated immune response is induced in the node, this deeper cortical tissue balloons right out and forms *paracortical nodules*.

The Spleen and Peyer's Patches

Lymph nodes are widely distributed around the body and constitute the most important source of antibodies in man. Another large organ of antibody production, however, is the spleen. This organ is evolutionarily older than the lymph nodes, and it has many functions. Several of these need not concern us greatly here. The spleen clears worn out red cells from the bloodstream and destroys them. It is also a factory for red cells, granulocytes, and the small "platelets" which help in blood clotting. In some species, such as the dog, the spleen is an important reservoir of blood. When a special need arises, its capsule can contract and discharge quite a lot of stored blood into the circulation. This is not a prominent feature of spleen function in man. In the lower fish, the spleen developed a lymphoid component which became more and more prominent and accounts for perhaps half of the volume of the mammalian spleen. This area, full of the whitish lymphocytes, is called the "white pulp" in contrast to the "red pulp," which contains blood and red cells in the process of destruction. The white pulp of the spleen is much like the cortex of the lymph node. However, there is one important difference. Foreign material arrives not by the lymph but by the arterial blood. The spleen is thus swollen in cases of blood poisoning. For the immunologist, it is the most important organ of antibody production when an injection of antigen is given directly into the bloodstream, for example, into a vein. Like the lymph node cortex, the spleen white pulp contains lymphoid follicles, but it does not contain typical postcapillary venules. The spleen red pulp is not really very similar to the lymph node medulla, and its structure need not concern us. However, it does have cords which contain most of the antibody-forming cells that develop after an antigen injection.

Literally billions of microorganisms inhabit our intestinal tracts. If any part of the intestine ruptures, for example the appendix, serious peritonitis results. The intestinal microorganisms thus possess the capacity to cause infections if they enter body tissues. Cells synthesizing IgA can be seen as a prominent component of the wall of the intestine. Another defense mechanism against intestinal invaders is constituted by a special population of lymph cell aggregates, termed Peyer's patches. These are very similar to lymph nodes. They are patches of lymphoid tissue actually embedded in the wall of the intestine, lying between the inner lining mucous membrane and the outer muscular coat. Peyer's patches do not have afferent lymphatics. Drainage is from the intestine itself. They do possess efferent lymphatics in the usual way. One particularly prominent feature of Peyer's patches is the presence of large lymphoid follicles with highly active germinal centers. This indicates that in normal health Peyer's patches are under constant antigenic barrage. This is not due to the entry of large numbers of living bacteria. Usually the integrity of the intestinal mucous membrane and the presence of intestinal antibodies prevent living bacteria from getting that far. It is probably the result of the entry of only partially digested bacterial breakdown products. Not surprisingly, the content of cells specialized for IgA production is very high in Peyer's patches.

The Thymus and the Bone Marrow

There remain two organs with which we will finish the anatomy lesson. These are our schools for lymphocytes, the thymus and the bone marrow. Neither is a battleground where antigen and lymphocyte meet. Rather, these are the factories for lymphocyte production and export. The thymus is covered fully in the next chapter. The bone marrow is that tissue which fills up the hollow spaces in bones. Most people know about the insides of long bones, such as the thigh bone. In fact, this type of bone marrow contains mostly fat. The more important part of the marrow is in the crevices and hollows which exist inside the ends of the long bones, the bones of the spine, and the pelvis. This marrow is colored red and is a great cell factory. Red cells, granulocytes, monocytes, and blood platelets are all made here. We now also know that the bone marrow is the source of many cells which, at a later stage of their maturation, become lymphocytes.

Thus a bird's-eye view shows us how diversified the body's defense system is. The circulating blood phagocytes are a mobile pool of first-line defenders. The all-purpose units of defense are the lymph nodes. Special defense forces for blood-borne invaders and intestinal microbes are the spleen and Peyer's patches. The source of raw recruits is the bone marrow; the military training school is the thymus. You may well wonder how, with this elaborate system, you can ever catch a cold or contract measles. It may be wise to recall that nature is not only on your side. She allows the viruses and bacteria as much right to exist as her proudest known achievement—man. The same forces of mutation and selection that have given man his lymph nodes are constantly at work in the microbial world; as hosts improve their defense methods, so parasites develop new characteristics allowing them to survive despite the immune apparatus. Just at the moment, man appears to be winning the struggle. Vaccination and antibiotics have tilted the scales in his favor. Yet the threat of the emergence of more virulent mutants can never be forgotten. Should these arise, we must at once identify them as we did with Asian flu in 1957. Constant vigilance provided by the human brain, combined with a sturdy defense system provided by evolution, should cope with most potential epidemics.

Lymphocyte Recirculation

Anatomy lessons tend to be static and rather boring, but the immune system is nothing if not dynamic. Lymphocytes love to circulate round the body, some traveling more extensively, some being relatively more sessile. Many lymphocytes are extremely long-lived, staying in their resting state for months or years if not hit by an antigen capable of triggering them. Lymphocytes have learned a clever way of getting round. They leave lymph nodes by the efferent lymphatic and finally pour into the bloodstream. They must "know," however, that their "best chance" of finding an antigen to stimulate them may be in a lymph node that has captured antigen. They therefore use the postcapillary venule of the lymph node cortex as a convenient escape hatch to reach the lymph node again. At any time, lymph node sections will show crowds of small lymphocytes in the lumen of these venules and squeezing their way through the walls into the lymph node. The lymphocytes may leave again by the efferent vessel and repeat the cycle.

We have mentioned scientists' propensity to work by building models. At the moment, the great vogue in cellular immunology research is to work with pure cell suspensions triggered by antigens in test tubes. The process of teasing these cells out of spleens or lymph nodes of course completely destroys the beautiful internal architecture and specialized microenvironments which nature has devised for the optimal functioning of the cells. It remains a great and unconquered challenge to reintegrate the precise knowledge gained through the reductionist approach into a "real life" setting. Those relatively few immunologists who work on the function of germinal centers, mechanisms of lymphocyte homing and traffic, or the architecture of the spleen as revealed by the electron microscope deserve thanks for continuing this difficult struggle.

8

SCHOOLS
FOR LYMPHOCYTES

THE 1960s witnessed a tremendous expansion in our understanding of the thymus, the first of our schools for lymphocytes. When I was a medical student studying physiology in 1950, so little was known about this organ that it warranted a scant half-page in most textbooks; this situation did not change greatly over the next few years. By the mid-1960s, so much new information had accumulated that three large international scientific symposia were held on the thymus in successive years, and several massive books were published. The history of this knowledge explosion speaks volumes about the way in which science develops. Since it is very intimately connected with The Walter and Eliza Hall Institute (the Australian research institute where I work), I propose to relate it in some detail.

The thymus is an organ of substantial size lying in the front of the chest just beneath the breastbone. It is sometimes referred to as the sweetbread. On microscopic examination it consists of a cortex (or shell) and medulla (or inner core). Both of these contain many lymphocytes, but these are much more densely packed in the cortex. In fact, the cortex is over 98 percent lymphocytes, with a few specialized reticular cells and a fibrous framework making up the rest. The medulla contains, as well as lymphocytes, considerable numbers of specialized cells that are called thymic medullary epithelial cells. It had been known for a long time that the size of the thymus varies greatly with age, and a detailed study of this in man was carried out in Germany in the 1930s. In fact, the thymus is a large, well-developed organ at birth. It then grows and reaches a maximum size around puberty. Subsequently, it slowly gets smaller again, and it can be quite tiny in advanced old age. One interesting thing about the thymus at any age is that it shrinks very rapidly if a person is seriously ill or subjected to great physical stress. Any long, debilitating illness tends to make the thymic cortex quite small. This feature of thymic behavior, which is still not well understood, led to some grave misconceptions in the early part of this century. Pathologists, whose job it is to study diseased organs and tissues, were really familiar with the thymus only through autopsy studies. Naturally, most people who die have had some preceding illness, frequently of long duration. Therefore most people who come to autopsy have small, shrunken thymuses. This caused many doctors to think that such small thymuses were normal; when people died suddenly from an accident or an unknown cause, and were found to have a thymus much larger than the usual postmortem specimen, these were frequently mistakenly regarded as abnormal. The phrase "status thymicolymphaticus" was coined and represented essentially a nonexistent disease! A little more was known about the thymus in mice than in man. Some inbred strains of mice are very prone to develop leukemia. It is possible to prevent some forms of leukemia from starting by removing the thymus in early life.

The modern era of thymus research really began in 1956 with the work of Dr. Donald Metcalf at The Walter and Eliza Hall Institute, who was trying to find out more about leukemia of lymphocytes in mice. He observed that the serum of leukemic mice and also of human leukemia sufferers contained something which stimulated a heightened level of lymphocytes in the bloodstream when injected into newborn mice. This factor was termed "lymphocytosis-stimulating-factor," or LSF. Closer study revealed that LSF was also present in normal mice but in much smaller quantities, and that it was made by the thymus. LSF was thought to be a regulator of the rate of lymphocyte production. Raised levels might be one of the factors leading to leukemia.

The next major step forward, in 1961, was taken by another colleague, Dr. J. F. A. P. Miller, then working at the Chester Beatty Research Institute in London. Dr. Miller was also interested in leukemia in mice. As part of an experiment which he was performing on the effects of the thymus on leukemia, he had to devise a surgical method of removing the thymus from newborn mice on the first day of their life. If you have ever seen a newborn mouse, which is less than an inch long and weighs about one gram, you will appreciate what a delicate surgical feat that was! The operation of taking out the thymus is called thymectomy, and if it is done on a newborn animal, it is termed a neonatal thymectomy. Long experience with adult thymectomy had shown that this was not followed by any obvious or dramatic ill-effects. If the mice got over the initial shock of the operation, they lived quite healthily for many months. The results in neonatally thymectomized mice were quite a surprise. They grew poorly, were runted and sickly, and at two or three months of age they usually died. This wasting disease could be prevented by grafting a thymus back into the animal. So, clearly, the thymus had some function that was vital to the healthy early development of the animal. When Dr. Miller examined some of the mice at autopsy, he found that the lymph nodes and spleen were very shrunken. This alerted him to the possibility that the mice might have a poorly functioning immune system. Therefore, he performed skin graft tests. These indicated a very severe impairment indeed of the cellular immune response. In fact, all

T cell functions were low, and, as antibody production to most antigens depends on helper T cells, humoral immunity was also impaired.

Dr. Miller's discovery created great excitement when it was reported at a conference in Italy in 1961 because, until that time, there had been no indication that the thymus could influence antibody mechanisms. His study showed that although the thymus did not itself form antibodies, it played a crucial part in the development of the immune system. It was a clear example of the reaction between chance observation and the prepared mind, which so frequently is at the root of major advances. Dr. Miller could so easily have said: "Look at those poor, runty mice; they'll be no good for anything," and turned his thoughts to other experiments. Instead, he realized that the least expected experimental result can be the most exciting, and should be followed up in a logical way.

Another facet of science is illustrated by this phase of thymus research. Somehow, great discoveries are frequently made almost simultaneously and quite independently in two or three laboratories in different parts of the world. There was nothing in Dr. Miller's experiment on neonatal thymectomy that required expensive equipment, and there is no real reason why it could not have been done years earlier, but no one had tried it. In 1961, quite independently and motivated by totally different reasons, another group in America also embarked on a study of neonatal thymectomy. Dr. R. A. Good of the University of Minnesota had come to have an interest in the thymus, both through clinical studies and comparative physiology. He encouraged his associates, Drs. O. K. Archer and J. C. Pierce, to develop a technique for neonatal thymectomy in the rabbit, with a specific view to testing the subsequent effects on the development of immune capacity. Archer and Pierce published their results in 1961, almost simultaneously with Miller. Unfortunately, it did not prove feasible to do the operation until the rabbits were five days old, and the immune defect which resulted when the operation was done at five days was not very marked. Within months of the publication of these two studies, numerous scientists were able to confirm the basic finding in a number of animal species and test systems.

Lymphocyte Differentiation within the Thymus

The thymus is thus the school and factory for T cells. The story is not quite this simple, however. The thymus itself receives an inflow of cells, of a very primitive and undifferentiated nature. As early as the eleventh day of fetal life in the mouse and about eight weeks of fetal life in the human, one can see these primitive cells crawling into the thymus. Previously these precursors had been resident outside the main body of the embryo in an area known as the yolk sac. The precursor cells are acted upon by one or more hormone-like molecules made by the thymic epithelial cells. One such hormone, thymopoietin, has been purified and its amino-acid sequence has been determined. At very low concentrations, it encourages precursors to switch on the genes needed to make the molecules and cell surface receptors characteristic of a T lymphocyte—for example the Thy-1 antigen mentioned in Chapter 4. Two other hormone-like agents are at a more preliminary, partially purified research stage. These, thymosin and thymin, may act at different stages of the differentiation pathway. Clearly the conversion of a precursor to a T cell is a multistage and complex process, and the presence of multiple inducer molecules is thus to be expected. Though thymopoietin can readily be detected in the circulation, it is probable that the multiple influences needed for correct thymic differentiation require the actual physical proximity of the epithelial cell making the hormone-like inducers and the differentiating thymus cells.

The inflow of precursor cells is not a once-and-for-all event in early embryonic life. In fact, there is a constant slow renewal of the thymic dividing cell population by an inflow of precursor cells. If a thymus is heavily irradiated and all its lymphocytes die, it will soon be repopulated by new cells slipping in from the bloodstream.

Life would be much simpler if I now could declare that all the T cells, once mature, promptly left the thymus and took their place in the anatomical battlegrounds (lymph nodes, spleen, Peyer's patches, etc., which together constitute the *secondary lymphoid organs*), joining the recirculating T cell pool. It certainly is true that many cells do just that. However, there is also much lymphocyte death in the thymus, and some workers have estimated that perhaps the majority of thymocytes die locally without ever leaving. Strange school indeed that murders its pupils! The puzzle may be partly explained by realizing that there are two streams of lymphocyte development in the thymus, with two sets of cells emerging. The one set possesses relatively little Thy-1 antigen, leaves promptly when mature, and behaves immunologically like self-respecting T lymphocytes should do. The other set has a very high concentration of Thy-1, appears on appropriate adoptive transfer to have no immunological function, and, though a few high Thy-1 cells leave and settle in the spleen, many certainly die before leaving. It is this second population which is at the root of our as yet unsolved dilemma.

The Contribution of Nudes to Immunology

No, I am not about to substitute pornographic analogies for the bloodthirsty military ones used so far; nor am I about to become an art critic. I am just going to write about nude mice! Some years ago, a genetic defect was discovered which, if possessed in a double dose, causes mice to be born which grow up totally lacking hair and without a thymus. In fact, a tiny thymus does develop in embryonic life but it fails to promote lymphocyte development and shrivels up. These mice have been extremely valuable research tools not only because they are provided by nature—and therefore the investigator is saved from having to perform the tricky neonatal thymectomy operation—but also because their defect in functional T cells is more complete. When the thymus is surgically removed at birth, there has already been time for quite a few T cells to slip out of the thymus in the last four days of embryonic life. These exist in the secondary lymphoid organs, get acted upon by antigens, multiply, and constitute a small, ineffective pool of peripheral T cells of just enough nuisance value to prevent experiments from being really clean. The nude mouse has provided a good bit of the information which we possess concerning T and B cell functions.

The Results of Adult Thymectomy

One of the reasons that the crucial role of the thymus in immunity was not discovered earlier is that its removal in adult mice or humans is not followed by any dramatic effects on the immune system. We now know that the adult thymus does continue to pump out new T cells and export them to the peripheral T cell pool, at least until the cortex atrophies late in life. However, for most practical purposes, the already existing pool of T cells in the adult is sufficient to maintain good T cell function for quite a while. In the mouse, if one waits six to nine months after adult thymectomy (a period representing about a quarter of the natural life span of the mouse, which is two to two-and-a-half years), serious immune deficiencies are noted. The peripheral T cells, though long-lived, are not immortal and do require slow, gradual renewal. Interestingly, in man, where adult thymectomy is sometimes performed because of tumors or other disease in the thymus, no immune defects have been reported, even though they have been looked for. Arguing by extrapolation, one might have to wait 20 years or longer for these to show up. Another possible explanation is that thymic removal may not have been quite complete. I suspect, however, that the real reason is that the peripheral T cell pool is given enough jolts by various antigens entering over this very long time span to fire a good proportion of the total repertoire into division, thereby rejuvenating the pool. We will look at this more closely in Chapter 11.

In the mouse, not all the T cell subsets are affected equally by adult thymectomy. In fact, the Ly 1^+, 2^+, 3^+ cells fall off in numbers rather rapidly. At this stage, it is not clear to what extent this is because such cells are essentially short-lived, and to what extent because they convert or mature into Ly 1^+, 2^-, 3^- or Ly 1^-, 2^+, 3^+ cells.

Birds, Bursas, and B Cell Birth

The thymus as the producer and exporter of T cells is, despite some of the complexities we have dwelt on, a simple discovery. But what of B cells? Unfortunately, the situation here is not nearly so clear-cut in either man or mouse. However, by a quaint quirk of evolution, the humble chicken has come to our rescue and told us that, in all probability, the fundamental rules for B cell birth are similar to those for T cells. It turns out that birds have, as well as a thymus, another thymus-like lymphoid organ called the *bursa of Fabricius*. This is located near the cloaca, the egg-laying orifice. In the chick embryo, it has been shown that precursor cells penetrate into the tiny, rudimentary bursa a day or two after they first enter the thymus, and, within the bursal environment, massive multiplication and gradual conversion to B cells takes place. Very recently the hormone *bursopoietin*, capable of converting primitive cells into cells with some B cell characteristics, has been described. Starting a few days before hatching, the bursa exports B cells at a great rate and sends them to the spleen and elsewhere to form the peripheral B cell pool. Like the thymus, the bursa is maximally active in young life and atrophies later.

Search as one might, one cannot find an organ like the bursa in mammals. All sorts of strange organs, such as the tonsil, Peyer's patches, even the appendix, have enjoyed brief, glamorous periods of intense scrutiny as possible bursal equivalents. Only in the past two or three years has something like a consensus been reached about what is going on. Bursal function is the production of inducers that persuade more primitive cells to differentiate towards the B cell lineage; and extensive multiplication of such cells is followed by seeding out to secondary lymphoid organs. In the mammals, these functions are diffused rather than sharply localized, and moreover occur in organs that also have quite different functions. The first site of bursal-like activity is in the fetal liver. In the adult, the mass production of new B lymphocytes occurs chiefly in the bone marrow and to a lesser extent also in the spleen, but *not* in the lymph nodes. It is not sure whether the bone marrow itself is making a bursopoietin-like hormone. While this would be the simplest solution, it is also possible that this is produced elsewhere and acts at a distance. Indeed, it is not at all clear how close the analogy between the bursa and the bone marrow really is. What is clear is that B cell neogenesis is much more diffused or multifocal in the mammal, not as vitally dependent on one geographical location. For example, when the bone marrow of a mouse is destroyed, more B lymphoneogenesis takes place in the spleen.

The convenient shorthand description "B lymphocyte" therefore stands equally for "bursal equivalent" or "bone marrow-derived" lymphocyte.

Neither the bursa in the bird nor the bone marrow in the mammal are significant sites of antibody production. Their job is to produce the cells that will be able to form antibodies after suitable triggering by antigens. It is convenient to refer to these schools for lymphocytes (thymus, bursa, bone marrow) as *primary* lymphoid organs, in order to distinguish them from the *secondary* lymphoid organs which trap antigens and provide the opportunities for mature lymphocytes to interact with them. This is depicted in Figure 8–1.

In the case of both bursa and bone marrow, the appearance of surface Ig is a rather late event in the B cell maturation process. It occurs after the last mitotic division of the "pre-B" lym-

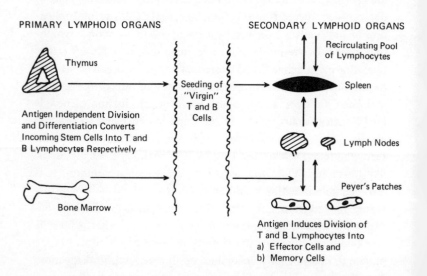

Figure 8–1.   Primary and secondary lymphoid organs.

phocytes, increasing amounts appearing progressively over about two days. The very young or newly formed B cells first display only IgM, as we have already noted in Chapter 4. The newly emerging B cells display interesting properties, as we shall see in Chapter 12.

Primary Lymphoid Organs and the Generation of Diversity

We have discussed in Chapter 5 the fact that different lymphocytes bear different receptors, each cell bearing only one unit of the recognition repertoire. There is thus immense diversity among lymphocytes. Where and what is the generator of diversity? There has been much speculation that this process, be it mutational or one of programmed differentiation, occurs in the primary lymphoid organs, where the massive and rapid multiplication would certainly provide opportunity. There are really two aspects of this problem, which we can take up most precisely for the B cell, the receptors of which are better understood. First, the cell must "decide" which of its V region genes (and it certainly possesses a set, though the dimension of this is not known) it will switch on. Secondly, for the majority of scientists who believe there must be some somatic process of genetic change in the cells, we must ask how many divisions it would take, at various postulated mutation rates, to generate a completely diversified repertoire. We know that in the mouse a reasonably diverse B cell repertoire exists by day 18 of embryonic life, and the first identifiable pre-B cells appear in the fetal liver only six days before that. As mouse cells cannot divide faster than once every seven hours at a maximum, this would give time for only twenty or so sequential divisions, not a large number for any

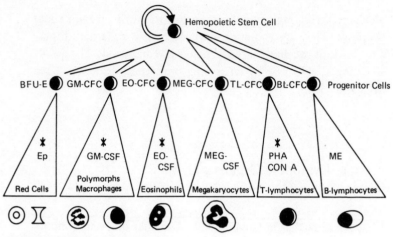

*Adapted for Culture of Human Cells

Figure 8–2.   The organization of the hemopoietic system.

Progenitor cells:	BFU-E	Burst forming unit-erythroid
	GM-CFC	Granulocyte-macrophage colony forming cell
	Eo-CFC	Eosinophil colony forming cell
	Meg-CFC	Megakaryocyte colony forming cell
	TL-CFC	T lymphocyte colony forming cell
	BL-CFC	B lymphocyte colony forming cell
Stimulus required for differentiation and multiplication in culture	Ep	Erythropoietin
	GM-CSF	Granulocyte-macrophage colony stimulating factor
	Eo-CSF	Eosinophil colony stimulating factor
	Meg-CSF	Megakaryocyte colony stimulating factor
	PHA	Phytohemagglutinin
	Con A	Concanavalin A
	ME	Mercaptoethanol

(Figure by courtesy of Drs. D. Metcalf and G. Johnson, The Walter and Eliza Hall Institute.)

conventional mutational process. However, as we do not know the molecular mechanism of somatic diversification, it is fruitless to speculate too far.

To this point, we have used the word "precursor cell" rather glibly to refer to the cells which migrate to thymus, bursa, or fetal liver and there are acted upon to differentiate into T or B lymphocytes. In fact, there are different hierarchies among these precursor cells as well, and a great deal of research has been done on them. There is a pool of ultimate precursors, or stem cells, first generated in the mouse very early in intrauterine life and located in the blood islands of the yolk sac, which are totipotent as far as blood is concerned. They possess the capacity to develop into any one of the many different blood cells. The term *hematogenous stem cell* should be used exclusively for such totipotent cells, a pool of which persists even in adult life, mainly in the bone marrow. However, these stem cells do not commit themselves to one pathway of differentiation all in one jump. Rather, perhaps a little like a medical student, they become specialists by stages. First they must "decide" whether to go towards the cell which is the common ancestor of red cells and the other white cells. Then, they act according to the schema shown in Figure 8–2. As far as lymphocytes are concerned, some recent work suggests that cells destined to wander into the thymus and to initiate T cell formation are already specialized before they enter the thymus. For example, in the nude mouse there appear to be cells with certain surface markers that suggest they are pre-thymic cells, waiting only for thymopoietin and the other inducers to act on them. The nomenclature in this field of hematology badly needs revision, but this will have to wait until the new concepts in Figure 8–2 have gained more general acceptance.

Perhaps it is reassuring that there are so many facets of the schools for lymphocytes requiring more research. The recent history of work on the thymus illustrates well a basic pattern in scientific research. At first there is darkness. Then a door suddenly opens—a shaft of bright light enters. It illuminates directly one shining piece of knowledge. But, as eyes take time to become adapted so that the whole room can be seen with just the shaft of light, so scientific data must gradually and painstakingly be accumulated so that not only the central fact, but its place in the total setting of knowledge in the field, can emerge. The first breakthrough brings an excitement beyond compare. Its full exploitation means years of hard and often tedious work. It is a judicious combination of the former and the latter that sets the seal on a person's scientific creativity.

9

TRIGGERING THE LYMPHOCYTE

THE CHEMISTRY of the body is under a myriad of delicate controls. The most central tasks, such as the digestion of food or the burning of glucose to yield the energy which drives the muscles, all require the concerted, sequential action of a series of enzymes, the cell's catalysts. These seem always to be present in the right concentration at the right place and at the right time. In fact, every cell is a masterpiece of chemical engineering. In the case of an immune response, we are also looking at an engineering problem and at an elaborate system of control loops. Whatever may be the situation in model systems, in real life the triggering of a lymphocyte never involves just one single cell, but rather a complex series of interactions between cells. Nor is the commonly used term really apt, because the action of an antigen on an immunocyte is not just like pulling the trigger of a gun at one instant in time. It involves sequential events spanning days. If we are to understand how antigen works in activating im-

mune responses, we have to strive to approach the issues both at
the level of the single cell and in terms of overall control. This
will be our task in the next two chapters.

The Meaning of Lymphocyte Activation

The lymphocyte comes out of school as a wandering but metabolically rather inactive cell. It has stopped dividing, and performs just enough work to keep it moving round the tissues,
which it does at a much slower rate than the phagocytic cells,
but very diligently nevertheless; and to maintain its component
parts, and particularly its surface receptors, in good working
order. When its watchfulness is "rewarded" through encounter-
ing an antigen with which its receptors will fit, the process of
activation *may* (not *will!*) begin. This involves a physical enlargement of the cell as it forms the new cytoplasmic factories
which it will need. New proteins and nucleic acids are made.
RNA synthesis, never at a complete standstill, accelerates considerably. Following a latent period of eight hours or longer,
DNA synthesis, which had stopped completely in the nondividing cell, begins again. This indicates that the cell is about to
double its DNA, making an exact copy of all the coded information, prior to dividing into two cells. These divisions are sequential, one cell going to two, two to four, four to eight, and so on,
until various feedback loops come into play. Simultaneously, but
at a rate depending on particular circumstances, the cells begin
to pour out their specialized products—antibody if it is a B cell,
helper or suppressor factors if it is a helper or suppressor T cell,
and so forth. The nature of the product depends not on the
antigen but on the properties of the cell. If the stimulated B cell
has a receptor specific for measles virus, its progeny will pour
out anti-measles antibody. It is predestined for that task and the
antigen serves only to unlock the potential within.

The creation of this army of specialized and highly active effector immunocytes is not the only result of the activation process. There is also the formation of *memory cells*, lymphocytes which revert to the nondividing state and ensure that a more active response occurs on second exposure to an antigen. At present we do not know whether these memory cells are "retired" effector cells or a separate segment of differentiation.

If circumstances are arranged artificially so as to circumvent physiological control processes, individual clones of immunocytes continually driven by antigens can get to be very large, hundreds of thousands or millions of cells in size. In most acute infections and immunizations, however, a more normal clone size might be in the hundreds or thousands.

Biochemical Events in Lymphocyte Activation

Antigens are not the only agents which can trigger lymphocytes. In fact, nearly all of the work on the early biochemical events of activation has been performed using model substances, accidentally discovered some years ago to have the property of switching on lymphocytes. In contrast to antigens, which switch on only those lymphocytes with receptors for that antigen—a very small fraction of the total pool—these model activators can turn on all the lymphocytes of a particular class, regardless of the specificity of the receptor. The most extensively used artificial activators (or *mitogens*, as they cause mitosis) have been substances extracted from plant seeds, such as those which go by the abbreviated names of PHA and Con A, which turn on T cells; or bacterial extracts, such as one termed LPS, which turn on B cells. Mitogens have been described which turn on only given subsets of the major classes.

These mitogens do not bind preferentially to the specialized receptors for antigen on the lymphocyte surface, e.g., the IgM of the B cell. Rather, they have the property of sticking to a wide variety of proteins, and we do not know which of these is important in the triggering process. One characteristic which all the commonly used mitogens share is that they are highly multivalent; they adhere to the cell by multiple binding sites per molecule.

Knowledge gained from studies of cell activation in nonimmunological systems has revealed that stimulators of dramatic changes in a cell's behavior frequently exert their action by causing the formation of molecules called cyclic nucleotides. The most important of these are called cyclic AMP and cyclic GMP. They act as the cell's internal messengers. They can cause activation or repression of specific genes. For example, many hormones act by raising cyclic AMP levels inside a cell, and so do some drugs. The detailed mechanism of this is quite tricky. It begins with the hormone or other inducer fitting to a specific receptor site on the cell membrane. This union causes a slight change in shape in the receptor, leading to a new site being exposed. This important principle in molecular biology is called *allostery*. The new or allosteric site starts an enzymic chain reaction which leads on to cyclic AMP or cyclic GMP production.

The analogies with antigen or mitogen action are obvious, and changes in cyclic nucleotide levels in recently activated lymphocytes have been looked for. Results have been somewhat variable from laboratory to laboratory, but a surge of cyclic GMP production has been reported as the internal message for lymphocyte division. The fact that this can occur without the mediation of the receptor for antigen is interesting. There has been much speculation around the multivalency of the mitogens. This has suggested that processes of cross-linking of receptors, or dragging two or more receptors together, might somehow initiate the allosteric change required. More complex theories, involving disruption of the tethering mechanisms for cell surface molecules by having them all tied to a multivalent ligand, have been proposed for signaling. Despite intensive endeavors, there is no crisp answer yet. Some of these issues will concern us again in Chapter 13.

Cellular Interactions in Lymphocyte Activation

I noted above that a union of antigenic determinant and lymphocyte receptor may, but need not necessarily, initiate lymphocyte activation. In fact, it is only a certain rather specialized set of antigens, the so-called T-independent antigens, which have the property of triggering a B cell directly. These share characteristics with mitogens, particularly multivalency. For most antigens, collaborative interactions between the cell to be activated and other cells are necessary for triggering. This subject is most conveniently discussed separately for T and B cells. Let us deal first with B cell activation.

Helper T Cells and B Cell Activation

The T-independent antigens stimulate mainly IgM antibody production. For production of IgG, IgA or IgE by B cells, the participation and help of T cells is required. Experiments involving fractionation of cells from immunized animals and their reassembly in various relative concentrations either in tissue culture or in adoptive transfer experiments have shown us some of the subtleties of T cell help. The helper cell is antigen-specific. It must recognize the antigen against which the B cell is reacting. However, we have already noted that most antigens are *mosaics* of several antigenic determinants. It turns out that, in order to help the B cell, the T cell must recognize some determinant other than the one the B cell is recognizing. For example, consider a hapten-protein conjugate such as dinitrophenol (DNP) hooked onto egg white (ovalbumin or OA) as an antigen. To switch on an anti-DNP B cell response and get good anti-DNP IgG antibodies, one has to provide helper T cells that have been activated against OA, not DNP. This prompted the formulation of the hypothesis shown in Figure 9–1 that T lymphocytes presented antigens to B cells in some specially attractive way. It now seems more likely that the helper T cell secretes one or more soluble factors which stimulate the B cell. There would not necessarily be an antigen bridge, as shown in Figure 9–1, but a diffusible, stimulating message, as shown in Figure 9–2. A number of laboratories are working hard to determine the chemical nature of antigen-specific T cell factors. As well as these, there is a family of antigen-nonspecific factors released from activated T cells. These cannot by themselves trigger B

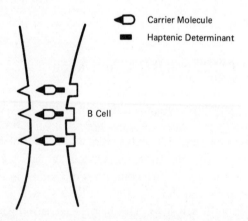

Figure 9–1.   T lymphocytes presenting antigens to B cells: the antigen bridge hypothesis.

cells but can increase the division rate and enlarge the size of appropriately triggered B cell clones.

As if this were not complicated enough, we must introduce a third cell type into the act, namely the macrophage. Its presence is essential in T-B collaboration, but we do not know exactly why. One plausible theory is that it is essential for the activation of helper T cells; another that T cell factors act *not* to stimulate the B cell directly, but rather to stimulate the macrophage to stimulate the B cell. All the relevant experimental findings are very new, and cell interaction obviously represents an area that will be more accessible for our third edition! Perhaps by then it will be 1984. . . .

Cell Interaction in T Cell Activation

This is even more intricate. First, it appears that T cells see antigens properly only when these are associated with a histocompatibility antigen (see Chapter 14), and this association normally occurs on the surface of a macrophage. The macrophage is essential for T cell activation in most circumstances. Second, even with effector T cells, be they ones helping B cells, or ones responsible for killing or suppression, an interaction between two categories of T cells, akin in principle to that just described for T-B interaction, and dependent on soluble factors, is involved. In other words, instead of T cells helping B cells, a set of Ta cells helps a set of Tb cells to get moving. In some respects, this has the flavor of a hall of mirrors; one wonders how many levels of interaction will eventually be discovered. Why T cells like to recognize histocompatibility antigens and conventional antigens in association with these is one of the most intriguing questions posed by recent research. It will be tackled in Chapter 14.

The reader may well ask why nature has designed such a

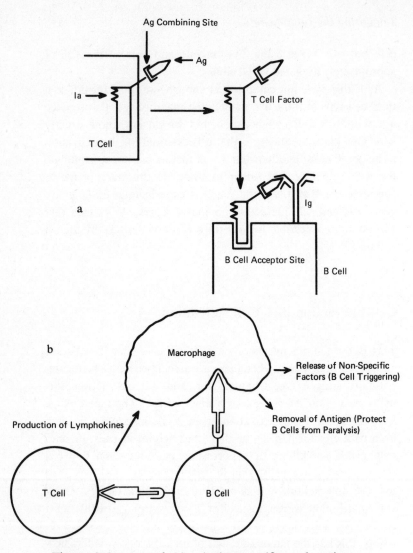

Figure 9–2. a) and b) Antigen-specific and antigen-nonspecific T cell factors. a) On this model, the T cell factor is seen as consisting of antigen (Ag), a T cell receptor for antigen, and the Ia molecule. The B cell is seen as having an acceptor site for Ia, and the presentation of antigen held jointly via the "cell interaction" Ia molecule and the Ig molecule is seen as providing the triggering

complex system for triggering. Would it not have been far more sensible just to have a receptor for an antigen on a cell, and a simple allosteric change leading to cyclic nucleotide production, in exact analogy to hormone action? Why bother with all this nonsense about cell interactions and T cell factors? The reason is tied up with the need for control. For one thing, if it is too easy to get an immune response rolling, the risk of forming antibodies to one's own tissues is correspondingly greater. For another, a "damped" system, with a responding cell set that can be helped or suppressed by sets of modulating cells gives far greater potential for regulation. Finally, it may just be that the molecules responsible for cell interaction represent a family that is older evolutionarily speaking than immunoglobulins, and was performing a task in some totally different kind of cell interaction. If so, it would have been natural for the later evolutionary adaptation of immune recognition to make use of this pre-existent potential in some way.

Antigen Distribution and Isotope Techniques

While many model experiments on triggering are done with lymphocytes in test tubes, nurtured by artificial growth media, the process really goes on in the secondary lymphoid organs such as the lymph nodes and spleen. These are rich in antigen-

---

stimulus. b) On this model, the T cell is seen as producing pharmacological molecules known as lymphokines, some of which activate the macrophage to produce its own specific B cell triggering factors. Some workers, notably Dr. G. Mitchell of The Walter and Eliza Hall Institute, see another major role for the macrophage, namely the removal of excess antigen, thus saving B cells from immunological paralysis.

trapping cells of various kinds. It is possible to mark antigens with radioactive isotopes and to follow their distribution and trapping within the body following injection. Radioactive isotopes are changed atoms made in a cyclotron or other nuclear reactor; occasionally they are found in nature. They have the property of disintegrating, and in the process giving off electrons, gamma rays, beta particles, or other forms of radioemission. Though the disintegration of each particular atom is a random affair, there are rules governing the radioactive disintegration rate of the whole population of atoms. Thus, the time it takes for half of the atoms of a particular isotope to decay can be accurately determined. This figure is called the "half-life" of the isotope. In biological studies, the half-life of most isotopes in common use varies from several hours to 5,000 years.

The key advantage of radioisotopes in biological research is that detection methods of such great sensitivity are available so that the presence of only a tiny trace of the radioactive material can be detected. Normally, the energy of the disintegrations, greatly amplified electronically, registers on a radioactive counter. An even more sophisticated way of detecting the presence of an isotope, and one which has been widely used in immunology, is shown in Figure 9–3. It is termed *autoradiography*. The principle of this method is that isotope in a tissue section or cell-smear preparation is detected by a photographic emulsion. The section to be examined for radioactivity is placed on a glass microscope slide. After suitable fixation, it is taken to a darkroom and covered with a thin layer of photographic emulsion. It is then stored away in a light-tight box. During this "exposure" period, a proportion of the radioactive atoms in the cells will decay. The emissions scatter randomly in all directions. Some of them go in the wrong direction; others may stop in the tissue itself and not reach the emulsion. Many, however, will enter the photographic layer and there cause a change in the silver halide crystals, resulting in the formation of a "latent image." Just as in regular photography, the latent image is con-

verted to precipitated silver grains by photographic development. Then the photo can be fixed and exposed to light just like
a snapshot. Clearly, the period of exposure of this microphoto
will be much longer than that used for photography. The actual
time will depend on the half-life of the isotope and, at times, the
patience of the scientist. For example, with an isotope such as
iodine[131], where the half-life is eight days, there is not too much
point in an exposure longer than 16 days. During the first eight
days, half the atoms fire off; during the next eight, half of the
remaining half. In other words, three-quarters of the silver
grains which would have formed in an infinite time have actually
formed in the 16 days. With the widely used isotope tritium
(^{3}H) it is a very different story. Here the half-life is 12 years.
Even the most dedicated scientist would not wait that long for
the result of an experiment! In such cases, exposure periods of
one to three months would be common.

Figure 9–3 shows what an autoradiograph might look like
under the microscope after development, fixation, and suitable
staining. The section shows profiles of five cells. Over the nuclei
of three of them a number of black dots can be seen. Radioactive
emissions have traveled from an isotope source in the nuclei,
and the "image" is the pattern of developed silver grains that
you see. Labeling can be much heavier, and in some experiments
confluent blackening over a cell, caused by the development of
all the silver grains present, may occur. If so, the detail of the
underlying cell's appearance will be obscured. Therefore, it is
more usual to adjust the exposure period of the autoradiograph
so as to obtain 10 to 30 grains over a cell. The basic principle
of autoradiography can also be applied to electron-microscopic
sections. Here, very thin layers of especially fine-grained emul-
sions must be employed. The silver grains which result are much
too small to see in the light microscope but show up readily in
the electron microscope.

Both light- and electron-microscopic autoradiography have
their special advantages. In the light microscope, and particu-

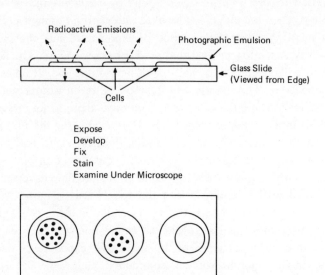

Developed Autoradiograph (Top View)

Figure 9–3. Detection by autoradiography of the presence of a radioisotope in a cell preparation. The black dots represent developed silver grains in the photographic emulsion overlying the section; they occur in two sorts of cells, as shown in Figure 9–5.

larly when whole cells rather than cell sections are examined, one can trace the presence of incredibly small amounts of material. In the most favorable case, about 10 molecules of an isotopically labeled substance in a cell could be detected. In the electron microscope, it is never possible to make the electron beam penetrate a whole cell, and very thin sections must be used. Perhaps two hundred sections would be taken through an individual cell. As it is rarely practicable to examine such a large number of sections of one cell, clearly much more isotope needs to be present for detection than in the case of the light-microscopic autoradiograph. Thus we lose some sensitivity. We make up for this by gaining much greater resolution, that is, a much more precise knowledge of where in the cell the isotopically labeled substance is actually located.

Capture of Antigen in a Lymph Node

Using a combination of light- and electron-microscopic autoradiography, we can gain exact knowledge of where the antigen goes. The purified antigen is first rendered radioactive. A convenient way of doing this is to hook on the isotope iodine[125]. This gives off suitably "soft" emissions for autoradiography, is readily counted in bulk in a radioactivity counter termed a scintillation counter, and has a half-life of 60 days, which is a reasonable exposure period. It is possible to inject less than a millionth of a gram of labeled antigen into an experimental animal and then follow its spread through the body.

In Figure 9–4, we see an example of a light-microscopic autoradiograph of a lymph node draining the site of injection of an isotopically labeled antigen. At low power, we can see that label has been concentrated in two areas of the node. The medulla is heavily labeled; most of the antigen is in the sinuses, but scattered labeled cells are also seen in the cords. In the cortex, the follicles are labeled, but the diffuse cortex is quite clear.

A more detailed view can be seen in Figure 9–5, which is a schematized version of what an electron-microscopic autoradiograph would show. Two entirely different processes are at work in the medulla and the follicle. In the medulla, the antigen is captured predominantly by macrophages. Some antigens prove relatively indigestible, and persist inside the phagolysosomes of macrophages for weeks or even months. In the lymphoid follicles, the antigen is captured by so-called dendritic cells. These do not engulf the antigen. Rather, the antigen remains attached

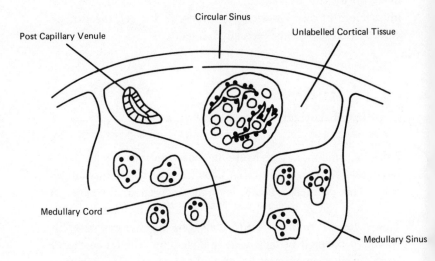

Figure 9–4. Low-power view of an autoradiograph of a
lymph node which has captured radioactive antigen.

to the surface of the cell, particularly to long, tentacle-like extensions which push their way between surrounding lymphocytes.
There are so many of these branching and intertwining dendritic
cell processes in a follicle that one can think of them as forming
a puff of cotton wool, the spaces of which are occupied by lymphocytes. Moreover, lymphocytes are not static but are in constant motion through this antigen-retaining web. Thus there is a
splendid chance for the surface of the lymphocytes to meet the
antigen stuck to a dendritic cell surface. The presence of some
antibodies in the blood and tissue fluids, as in a previously immunized animal, markedly favors follicular localization of the
antigen and therefore the surface persistence mode of trapping.

Recently, cells have been described which possess some of the
features of each of the two classical cell types, i.e., some engulf-
ment and some surface persistence. There is good reason to believe that it is the antigen on the cell surface of dendritic cells
and macrophages which provides the inductive stimulus for

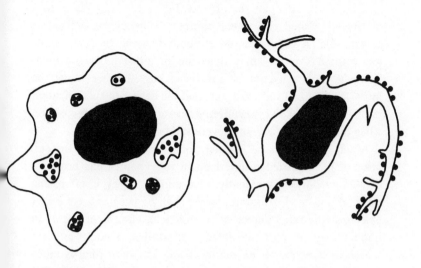

Figure 9–5. The two chief types of antigen-trapping cells in lymph nodes.

lymphocytes. This seems particularly likely for particulate antigens, which are very quickly cleared from the blood and lymph, and which really do not have much of a chance to encounter lymphocytes swimming there. It is probable that macrophages break such antigens into smaller bits, and re-expose the fragmented molecules on the cell surface, possibly in a constant, dynamic cycle.

Absence of Antigen from Antibody-forming Cells

Although it is probable that small amounts of antigen or antigen fragments enter at least a proportion of the ancestors of antibody-forming cells, autoradiographic study has shown that the majority of antibody-forming cells do not themselves contain antigen. Antigen begins the process, but in the later life history of the stimulated cell, there comes a stage when antigen is dispensable. A fully matured antibody-forming cell can do its job without even a single molecule of antigen being present inside it. This may not be surprising now that we know the importance of cell surface events and the degree of specialization implied by clonal diversification. It was an important observation when direct template theories were still being considered.

Much remains to be learned about antigen action. In fact, most of the knowledge described in this chapter has been accumulated only very recently. Our understanding is increasing daily, and as we learn more, so we shall be progressively better able to apply our discoveries to practical, clinical problems in immunology. In part, the intense effort that is going into research in lymphocyte activation at the time of writing is motivated by the challenges, surprises, and puzzles inherent in cell interactions, and by the immense medical implications of learning how the trigger really works.

10

GROWTH CONTROL
IN TRIGGERED CELLS

IN THIS ERA of economic awareness, nearly everyone is familiar with the most fundamental of all scientific illustrations, the graph. In its commonest form, a graph plots changing company sales or profits against the passage of time. Such a telling manifestation of the company's welfare is this simple drawing that cartoonists have made it a part of everyday folklore. In fact, a scientific analysis of the graph, combined with certain other knowledge, can frequently reveal a great deal about the company as a whole.

In this chapter, we will be involved with the graph in Figure 10–1—the progressive rise and fall of the level of antibodies in the serum after the injection of a powerful vaccine. This graph has fascinated students of immunology for 50 years, and ever more detailed analysis has given us deep and precise insights into the cellular events of antibody production. It must be stated right at the outset that this figure is a stylized graph, and that many factors may act to alter the shape of the curve under particular experimental circumstances. Nonetheless, it describes most of the important features of the dynamics of antibody production. Note that the level of antibodies plotted on the left rises, not in an arithmetic, but in a logarithmic progression. That is, it goes not 1, 2, 3, 4, . . . , 10, but 1, 10, 100, . . . , 10^n. This is the usual way to express results in any system where rapid multiplication is at work. Note also that the baseline is not set at a zero level of antibodies, but rather at 0.01 μg/ml of serum (1 μg $=$ one millionth of a gram). This brings out an important point. It is never possible to claim that a serum sample contains no antibodies to a particular antigen. It is only possible to claim that (1) the sample contains no *detectable* antibodies with the method used, and (2) the method used is sufficiently sensitive to detect any amount greater than, say, 0.01 μg/ml. There may be a substantial "iceberg" effect in many curves of antibody production. We see the part of the iceberg which pokes above the water level of 0.01 μg/ml. We do not see the events of antibody production which may be occurring earlier but lead to levels in the serum of only, say, 0.001 μg/ml. This, for a long time, frustrated our attempts at understanding the earliest cellular events in an immune response. The graph shows a "latent period" after the injection of antigens, during which time no detectable antibodies appear in the serum. It should be understood by now that the actual length of this latent period is influenced by the sensitivity of the antibody-detection method. In most cases it varies between one and four days. Then follows a period of rapid rise in serum antibody levels. Often this is a straight line when a "semi-logarithmic plot," such as in Figure 10–1, is employed. The rise can be quite steep, with antibody levels doubling every eight hours, or even more quickly. This phase lasts from two to three days and then tapers off. In some systems, a transient fall in blood antibody levels follows early in the second week, with a rise later in the second week. The subsequent course of events is quite variable, but usually antibody

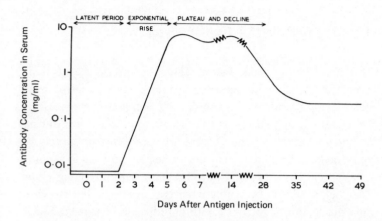

Figure 10–1. The rise and fall of serum antibody levels after a single injection of a powerful vaccine.

levels decline over the next few weeks. Frequently, a low residual level of antibodies can be detected for months, or even years, after a single antigen injection.

Obviously, these features of the antibody curve reflect the cellular events of activation and growth control in the lymphocyte population. The watchful B lymphocyte is not itself an antibody-former; it makes just enough IgM to replace the surface receptors as they are shed off from time to time. The latent period reflects the phase of antigen capture and processing, cell interaction, and the building of antibody-producing cytoplasm in the activated B cells. The logarithmic rise reflects repeated mitotic divisions, and the plateau and decline occur both because the antigen is gradually broken down and eliminated from the body, and because of some negative control loops. In discussing growth control, most of our examples will concern B cells but the important rules affect T cell clone growth just as much.

Regulatory Role of T Lymphocytes

It is clear that a major factor regulating the degree of clonal proliferation amongst activated lymphocytes is control by T cells. Using Ly markers, helper T cells outnumber suppressor T cells in the lymphoid tissues of normal animals, but it is difficult to know what this means as there are surely further subsets yet to be defined. One interesting role of helper T cells is to promote a switch in the class of Ig synthesis by a proliferating clone. Many clones begin by synthesizing IgM antibody, but switch to IgG production if provided with appropriate help from T cells activated to the carrier determinants of the antigen concerned. This switch interests geneticists, because it implies a transloca-tion of V region genes from μ constant region to γ constant region genes. There is no change in antibody-combining spec-ificity when this switch occurs—the V regions of both heavy and light chains are exactly as before. It is probable that this switch is in some way associated with germinal centers, the specialized structures already mentioned in Chapter 7. These contain an elaborate network of antigen-capturing cells, a large number of rapidly dividing B cells, and a small but definite con-tent of T cells. The development of germinal centers approxi-mately coincides with the switch to IgG production, and nude mice (lacking T cells) are grossly deficient in germinal centers and very poor at IgG antibody production. The ready avail-ability of antigens bound to dendritic cell surfaces and the presence of both T and B cells make the germinal center an attractive possibility as an anatomical site for T–B cooperation. A further interesting point is that germinal center cells them-selves produce few antibodies. The environment there promotes chiefly multiplication, and not so much differentiation. It is the B cells leaving germinal centers and migrating the short dis-tance to the medullary cords of lymph nodes or the red pulp of the spleen that actually develop into rapidly secreting plasma cells. Here, the microenvironment clearly favors specialization, with much less cell division.

The regulatory role of suppressor T cells is definitely important but not yet well understood. Factors favoring the development of suppressor cells include a high antigen dose, prolonged persistence (or re-administration) of the antigen, and avoidance of antigen trapping by macrophages. All of these conditions apply to the "self" antigens against which we certainly ought not to form antibodies, such as our own red blood cells or serum proteins. Suppressor cells might also be useful in limiting the amount of antibodies produced to constantly persisting antigens, such as those of bacteria that inhabit the intestine throughout life, as perfectly normal and in fact helpful companions or *symbionts*. In experimental situations, it is the balance between help and suppression which (together, of course, with the antigen dose) determines the amount of antibodies formed by a given number of B cells in a given time.

Negative Feedback by Antibodies

Very early in an immune response, it can be shown that tiny quantities of IgM antibodies first formed actually *help* the process of antibody formation; they provide a *positive feedback*, especially in experiments where only tiny quantities of antigen are used. This is probably because of improved antigen trapping and better follicular localization, as discussed in Chapter 9. Later in the response, a more important and more general phenomenon is noted, namely negative feedback by antibodies. It can be shown that the pre-injection of substantial amounts of antibodies into an animal can prevent an antigen from "taking." This fact was realized a long time ago. For example, babies who have acquired IgG antibodies to the common diseases like measles from their mother by transfer across the placenta are not given vaccines for three months or longer, permitting time for metabolic decay of most of the passively acquired antibodies. Negative feedback by antibodies works in two ways. First, the antibody covers up the antigenic determinants. This can be viewed as a kind of competition for antigen between freely circulating antibodies and the antibody receptor molecules on the lymphocyte surface. Unless the latter have a good chance of winning the competition, triggering cannot occur. Obviously large amounts of serum antibody will swamp the antigen and prevent it from finding the receptors. Second, it has been noted that soluble complexes of antigen and antibodies made with a slight excess of antigen (see Chapter 3), can efficiently stop lymphocytes from being triggered by antigen given in immunogenic form, e.g., as a bacterial particle. This is because the multivalent antigen-antibody complex is very efficient at jamming up the available B cell receptors.

Affinity Maturation in the Immune Response

We noted in Chapters 3 and 4 that the fit between an antigenic determinant and an antibody-combining site had to be viewed in quantitative terms, i.e., antibodies varied in affinity. In animals or people given repeated immunization, the affinity of the antibodies improves with time. Not only are more antibodies made, but they are of progressively better quality. This affinity maturation gives a good example of growth control in the immune system (Figure 10–2). When an antigen is first injected there is plenty of it around and many cells will be stimulated, both those that happen to have receptors with poor binding and those with high affinity receptors. As time goes on, antibodies are formed,

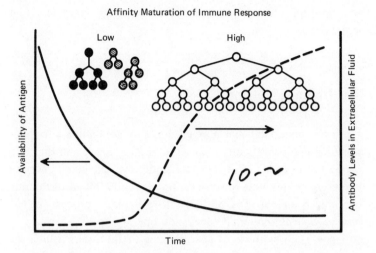

Figure 10–2.   Affinity maturation of the immune response. Early after antigen injection, antigen concentration is high and many clones, even those of low affinity, are stimulated. As antigen levels decline with time, only those clones with high affinity receptors manage to capture enough antigen and keep dividing.

and in the dynamic equilibrium situation that develops, those with the best-fitting determinants will compete most successfully for the residual antigen, and will therefore undergo the most divisions. In fact, in animals that have been frequently immunized, a few clones or even one come to dominate the picture. This is an example of the "survival of the fittest" rule, which seems to apply just as profoundly in the microcosm of an individual lymphoid system as it does in the macrocosm of the whole biological universe. There is one theory which holds that antigenically activated cells have a very high rate of mutation in Ig V genes, creating minor variants and speeding up affinity maturation, but this notion, which smacks somewhat of Lamarckism, has not yet gained many adherents. Affinity maturation depends on adequate T cell help, because without this the extensive multiplication of immunocytes required could not be maintained.

The Immune Network

We have mentioned that a given antibody-combining site, possessing a unique structure, can serve as an antigen, and that this is referred to as the *idiotype* of the antibody. Any given idiotype is present in minutely low concentration in the blood of the unimmunized animal. The normal self-recognition process, called *immunological tolerance*, does not operate for "sequestered" antigens, such as those of spermatozoa or the brain, which do not normally circulate in the blood or tissue fluids. Nor does it operate for idiotypes, again for reasons of molecular concentration. Therefore, when an idiotype is produced through normal immunization, the potential exists for anti-idiotype antibodies and T cells to be formed by the very animal being immunized. Through the same logic, anti-anti-idiotypes could occur, and we again see the "hall of mirrors" possibilities in the immune system. In fact, very recently, anti-idiotypic antibodies have been noted as a result of immunization. The immune system thus has properties of a network. If one thinks about anti-idiotypic antibodies, one will note that they have some of the properties of the original antigen—they combine with the same receptor that the antigen combines with (though not necessarily in exactly the same way). It has been shown clearly that anti-idiotypic antibodies can indeed stimulate both T and B cells. Conversely, anti-idiotype T cells possess the potential to kill T or B cells bearing that idiotype. Thus there are possibilities for both positive and negative feedback control. Only further studies will show whether these observations represent exotic laboratory curiosities or important elements of immune physiology.

Irradiation

Ionizing radiation such as X-rays or radioactive fallout from a nuclear bomb can cause severe damage to living cells. DNA molecules are particularly susceptible to irradiation-induced breaks in the gene strands. Though repair enzymes exist, there is a limit to the amount of damage which is compatible with later cell division. For this reason, dividing cells, which must duplicate their DNA as an essential event in mitosis, are especially susceptible to irradiation; and we have seen how important mitosis is in immunity. Moreover, some of the subsets of lymphocytes are susceptible to much smaller doses of irradiation than are needed to prevent division. They are destroyed, even though in a resting phase of the growth cycle, by a process called *interphase death*. Suppressor T cells are among this group. Irradiation with X-rays or gamma rays is a much used tool in immunology. For example, high dose irradiation can wipe out the whole of the lymphoid system of an animal, but leaves macrophages and dendritic cells in good shape; such animals can then be transfused with known numbers of various subsets of lymphocytes to determine their respective functions. Alternatively, the relative radioresistance of activated helper T or B cells can be employed to good effect. There are even circumstances where a low dose of X-irradiation can increase antibody formation, perhaps through selective killing of suppressor cells. Medically, the much-publicized importance of ionizing radiation lies both in its capacity to destroy blood-forming organs, hair follicles, intestinal epithelium, and other rapidly dividing cells at high dose; and the capacity for causing DNA breaks, and thus mutations, at low dose. Statistically, these carry risks for genetic malformations in the offspring of irradiated people, and a heightened cancer incidence in the people themselves. Fortunately, extreme precautions are now taken to minimize irradiation doses in diagnostic X-ray or radioisotope work. For all practical purposes, the risks from these are so minuscule as to be negligible.

Adjuvants

Adjuvants are substances that have been discovered through empirical observation to heighten immune responses. Among the most widely used in experimental work is Freund's adjuvant, a mixture of killed tubercle bacilli, mineral oil, an emulsifying agent, and the antigen in watery solution. The water-in-oil emulsion provides for a slow release of antigen, giving a kind of built-in booster effect. The dead bacteria, and particularly certain fatty molecules of the cell wall, provide a nonspecific stimulus to both lymphocytes and macrophages, the molecular basis of which is not yet known. Freund's adjuvant is too drastic for human use, but killed bacteria that are relatives of diphtheria or whooping cough have been tried, as has the tuberculosis-like BCG vaccine. In the human, adjuvants find their main role in attempts to boost immune defenses in cancer patients. An entirely safe and molecularly well-understood adjuvant would be important as an adjunct to ordinary killed vaccines as well, and the search for this continues.

Transfer Factor

In the human, it is possible to transfer the state of cell-mediated immunity from one person to another not only by injecting living cells but also by a cell-free extract. For example, if one person has had subclinical tuberculosis, and is tuberculin positive, a suitable extract of his or her white blood cells can be

injected into another person, and convert him from tuberculin
negative to tuberculin positive. Unfortunately, there is no really
reliable parallel to this finding in laboratory animals, and it has
proven difficult to determine what this phenomenon is all about
because of the obvious difficulties and constraints in research
on humans. The material transferring the T cell immunity has
been termed *transfer factor*. It is of low molecular weight, probably in the vicinity of 3,000, and has not yet been completely
purified. There is some doubt about just how specific for antigen
it really is, and the best guess at the moment is that transfer
factor represents a powerful but rather nonspecific way of
switching on T cells. Quite a lot of clinical work has been done
injecting transfer factor made from healthy people's blood into
people who show severe T cell deficiency. The latter can occur
either as an inherited defect or as a result of certain chronic
diseases, in which the T cell system almost ceases functioning.
How effective transfer factor really will prove in the overall
management of these conditions remains to be seen.

Decay of Immune Response

When the antigen-imposed drive to cell proliferation and differentiation comes to a halt, the shape of the antibody curve
depends on two things: (1) the life span of the mature antibody-
forming cells; and (2) the life span of the antibody molecules
themselves. Most antibody-forming cells are quite short-lived.
They secrete antibodies at maximal rate for two to four days
and then disappear. A significant minority, however, live for
much longer—weeks, months, or occasionally even years. We
do not know what determines how long a given mature antibody-
forming cell should survive. However, it is clear that the long-
lived variety of cell is quite important. It will continue to
synthesize antibodies long after the injection or infection which

caused its appearance. As the total number of long-lived antibody-forming cells is quite small, the antibody level in the serum may be relatively low. Yet it could still be sufficient to prevent a recurrence of some serious infection. The persistence of antibodies after some infections is lifelong. Some scientists believe this must be due to undetected re-exposure to the causative microbe, or perhaps to the microbe having gone "underground"—a virus gene living undetected inside a cell but still causing the formation of viral antigens. The rate of degradation of the antibody molecules themselves depends on the class of immunoglobulin. In rats, for example, about half of the IgG molecules formed at a given time will have been broken down by the body some six days later. In other words, the half-life is six days. IgM is a much less stable molecule. In the rat, its half-life is only 18 hours. In the human, the breakdown of antibodies is somewhat slower, IgG having a half-life of about two weeks. The disappearance of formed antibody molecules illustrates a very fundamental aspect of the behavior of living systems. Everything is in a constant state of flux: synthesis and degradation are delicately balanced; cells, structures, and compounds are made only to be broken down again. The only exception to this general rule is the magic DNA molecule, and even it is not quite as stable as was once thought, being subject to a certain amount of breakage and repair.

Control Loops in a Realistic Setting

Are the various control loops in growth of immunocyte clones of any practical importance? The answer is surely yes, as one of the finest recent advances in obstetrics has shown. When a woman with an Rh-negative blood group conceives a child by an Rh-positive man, the child's blood group may be Rh-positive.

This embryo's red blood cells are potentially antigenic in the mother. During her first pregnancy, nothing untoward will happen, as the amount of Rh-positive baby blood leaking through into her body will not be sufficient to cause a primary immune response. However, during labor the severe contractions of the womb will squeeze significant quantities of fetal blood into the mother. Some days after the baby is safely delivered, the mother synthesizes anti-Rh antibodies. When she conceives her second child, the child could be in trouble if it is also Rh-positive. The immunological memory function, which we will discuss fully in Chapter 11, gives the mother a heightened reactivity to Rh antigens. The tiny amounts of fetal blood which do leak across the placenta during pregnancy cause antibody formation in the mother. IgM antibodies are too big to cross back into the embryo. However, soon the mother's antibody-forming system switches to IgG antibody production. IgG molecules can cross the placenta and get back to the baby. Here they cause a severe anemia which is often fatal to the embryo. Once a woman has given birth to one affected child (the so-called Rh-baby) the chances are that every Rh-positive child that she carries will be progressively more and more seriously affected.

Now this whole tragic process can be prevented. Remember that Ig antibody has powerful negative feedback properties. If the mother, immediately after giving birth to her first (un-affected) child, is given a dose of anti-Rh IgG prepared from another human volunteer, antibody formation does not start in the mother. Thus, the next child is not affected. When it is born, she is given another dose of the passive anti-Rh antibody. Again, the negative feedback cuts in; the Rh antigen cannot "take" in her. As a result of the widespread use of this wonderful form of preventive medicine, the incidence of Rh disease has fallen dramatically in those countries that have used it widely. This is just one more example of the impact that theoretical studies of normal bodily functions can have on problems of disease.

In many respects, the immune response, with all of the cellu-

lar multiplication and tooling up that is required, is not ideal
to cope with the *first* infection by a very virulent microbe. This
may wreak its damage within two or three days of entry into
the body, and the patient may die despite the best efforts of the
lymphocytes. However, should recovery occur, the struggles of
the lymphocytes have not been in vain, because residual antibodies and cell-mediated immunity may last for life. Looked at
from the point of view of the microbe or parasite, the only way
these can make sure not to run out of susceptible hosts (and
thus die out) is either to mutate to a different antigenic pattern,
or to exist on some superficial part of the body such as the skin,
where the antibodies and cellular guardians are not so active.
These ecological considerations lead us on to the broader questions of immunological memory.

11

IMMUNOLOGICAL MEMORY

EVERY PARENT knows that an adequate immunization program involves not just one injection of a vaccine but one or more "booster" shots. To get a really good level of antibodies in the serum, it is often necessary to give two or more spaced antigen doses. If antibody levels in the blood are studied closely after both the first and the second vaccine injection, the curve will follow the pattern seen in Fig. 11–1. The second injection elicits the formation of far more antibodies than the first, even though the same dose of antigen has been used. The increase will frequently be tenfold, or even a hundredfold. This capacity for a heightened response on the second administration of an antigen is termed immunological memory, and the boosted reaction of the immune system is called a secondary response.

Immunological memory is specific for the antigen concerned. If we have two unrelated antigens, A and B, we can give an injection of A and four weeks later an injection of B. There will follow a primary response against A, and also a primary response against B. Provided the two antigens are of equal immunogenicity and are given in equal doses, the amount of anti-B formed will be neither more nor less than the amount

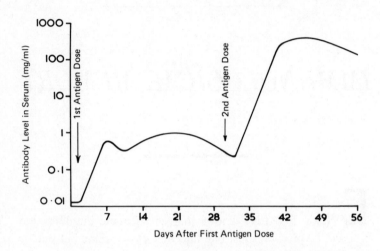

Figure 11–1. Kinetics of appearance of antibody after first and second doses of antigen four weeks apart.

of anti-A. For a booster reaction to ensue, the two injections must be of the same antigen or of two related ones.

The latent period before the rapid, logarithmic rise in antibody levels is generally shorter in a secondary response. In part this is due to a lesser "iceberg" effect, but in part it may also reflect the more rapid maturation of precursor cells. Another difference between primary and secondary responses is that the IgG antibody comes up much earlier in the secondary response. In fact, IgM and IgG tend to rise simultaneously, but IgG goes to much higher levels. Overall, IgG is the dominant antibody class in secondary responses.

Not all antigens demonstrate the memory phenomenon equally well. It is best shown up with antigens which cause practically no detectable primary response. This can be because of low inherent immunogenicity or because a very small dose is used. In such cases, a second "shot" will often cause surprisingly large responses. If an antigen already causes a substantial amount of antibody formation on first injection, the booster phenomenon may be of small degree and relatively short-lived. This is probably because negative feedback mechanisms set an absolute ceiling for immune responses. If the amount of antibodies formed on first challenge already approaches this ceiling, the secondary response will not appear dramatic.

The Cellular Basis of Immunological Memory

The key to understanding immunological memory lies in understanding clonal selection. For both T and B cells, each cell represents just one small word in the immunological dictionary. Suppose that a mouse has 10^9 lymphocytes, half T and half B. Suppose an antigen X comes along, and 10^5 cells bear receptors of sufficient affinity to X to be stimulated to divide. Because of diversity in affinity, not all will go through the same number of divisions, but let us say that the 10^5 anti-X cells divide five sequential times on the average. Each would then create a clone of $1\times2\times2\times2\times2\times2$ or 2^5 cells—that is, 32 cells. Some of these engage in immunological action (form antibodies, or engage in T cell help) and some revert to the resting growth state and become memory cells. Unfortunately, we are woefully ignorant both about the proportion of cells which do the latter, and about the relations between effector immunocytes and memory cells. For the sake of argument, let us say that 16 of the 32 cells become memory cells. Of course, these do not live forever, but they are certainly long-lived on the average, probably longer-lived than the "virgin" cells which gave rise to them. The same antigen X reintroduced a few weeks later thus encounters 1.6×10^6 anti-X cells. Moreover, the affinity of these is higher, on the average, than that of the virgin starting population, because high-affinity cells have given more children than low-affinity cells. So, there are more cells reactive to antigen X, and they are of better average quality. They will "see" the antigen present in lower concentration than will a virgin population. This is one factor leading to increased responsiveness of the system.

Immunology has few concepts which can survive unqualified, and there are complexities to the above simple picture. First, the persisting antibody will have effects on re-injected antigen X, more often harmful to the immune response but sometimes helpful. Second, some of the memory cells will be suppressor T cells, but an excess of these over helpers is achieved only by rather specialized regimens of immunization. Third, there are interesting inherent distinctions between virgin cells and memory cells just in the process of being worked out. These involve differences in surface receptors, susceptibility to mitogens, re-circulation characteristics, life span, and possibly even slight differences in size. Memory thus has aspects which make it impossible to describe by a simple number.

Germinal Centers and the Memory Function

Although proof is not at hand, it is likely that many of the memory cells generated by the body are formed in germinal centers. You will recall that these are rounded nests of big blast cells which develop in lymphoid follicles after an antigen has been deposited there. The sequence of events which follows antigen deposition can be studied by examination of histological sections taken from lymph nodes of animals killed at serial intervals after the antigen injection. Before any antigen comes along, follicles contain few, if any, blasts. Within about four hours after the injection of a powerful antigen, significant amounts have entered the follicle and become attached to dendritic cells. Follicular localization reaches maximum intensity in about one day. With less powerfully immunogenic antigens, follicular localization may not take place until much later. Within the first day or so after the antigen deposition, there is not much visible change in the follicle. However, soon thereafter significantly increased numbers of scattered blast cells appear; these represent antigen-reactive lymphocytes that have wandered into the follicle, have been locally stimulated, and start to divide. With a strong antigenic stimulus, little nests of four to twelve big blasts can be seen in follicles already two to three days after an antigen injection. As these divide, and as new antigen-reactive cells traverse the follicle, the number of blasts builds up. When the total number of cells in the nest reaches 100 or so, the term *germinal center* is applied to it. The heavier the antigenic stimulus, the bigger the germinal centers become. Repeated injections of antigen may be necessary to obtain maximal germinal center activity, and the biggest germinal centers contain thousands of blasts. Finally, however, there comes a stage when the germinal center cannot grow any more. Long before this stage has been reached, the germinal center is a powerful lymphocyte export factory. Though it is not possible to trace accurately the fate of germinal-center-born lymphocytes by direct techniques, a great deal of inferential and correlative evidence exists to suggest that many of them enter the lymph and finally the blood as long-lived, small, memory lymphocytes.

Original Antigenic Sin

This is the picturesque phrase which has been introduced to describe a situation first noted in regard to influenza virus infection. As we all know, the immunity conferred by a particular attack of influenza is not very good. This is partly due to the fact that flu is a superficial infection, the organisms multiplying in the mucous linings of the nose, throat, and upper respiratory tract, but not usually spreading through the bloodstream. Despite the valuable IgA molecule, one would not expect as solid immunity as for a virus like measles. Nevertheless, it has been proven that a flu attack or even an effective flu immunization, while by no means 100 percent protective, still significantly lessens the chances of being infected with the same flu strain over the next year or more. What happens, however, is that genetic changes occur in the most important flu virus antigens, and changed strains manage to elude the antibody screen put up by the body. In time, the total amount of immunity in the human population is so significant that an antigenic variant enjoys a great survival advantage, and rapidly becomes the dominant strain circulating between people. Mutation is the cause of minor antigenic changes that occur every year or so, and genetic recombination between human and animal flu viruses lies behind the major changes that come at intervals of a decade or more. In any case, there continues to be an *antigenic relationship* between the variant flu strains. They are not totally different from one another, as a flu virus would be from a polio virus. Rather, antisera which neutralize the old strain when diluted 1,000 times now neutralize the new strain only when diluted much less. Symbolically, one might think of the original strain as being antigenically A B C D E, a mutant strain as A B C D F, and a recombinant strain as A B G H I. Polio, of course, would be V W X Y Z.

Original antigenic sin means that the first flu attack exerts a steering force on all later immune responses to influenza. For example, individuals alive during the great influenza pandemic of 1918, when reinfected by the Asian flu, which first appeared in 1958, will make antibodies that neutralize swine flu better than Asian flu. Considering our alphabetical model, clonal selection explains that data well. Suppose that the person managed to retain 10 memory cells for every cell originally stimulated by the swine flu. Then, if the two strains are A B C D E and A B G H I respectively, the first infection creates a tenfold increase in A-reactive cells, B-reactive cells, and so forth for C, D, and E. When the second infection comes along, there will then be 10 anti-A and 10 anti-B cells for every G, H, or I reactive cell. No wonder the memory cells dominate the response that ensues.

It is likely that adult humans work on their immunological memory systems to a great extent, and that the repertoire of information contained among the immunocytes stimulated over the years by one of the many antigens encountered in normal life is very great. If this is so, there is almost no need for lymphoneogenesis in adult life in such long-lived animals as man, and this may account for the apparent innocuousness of adult thymectomy in man. The serum antibodies of adults contain an interesting fingerprint of past infections, and, as in many aspects of human life, past experience guides future actions.

We have not referred to the T cell in the above analysis, but it undoubtedly plays its role in original antigenic sin. In fact, memory carrier-primed T cells are a very important factor in ensuring a brisk memory IgG response. With one interesting exception to be mentioned in Chapter 14, all T cell phenomena show memory according to basically the same principles as B cells.

Epidemiology and Immunological Memory

Is immunological memory of basic importance to human health?
The answer to this question can be given quite unequivocally
from an examination of epidemiological data gathered in remote
Pacific islands and other isolated regions. There are by now
many well-documented examples of "virgin soil" epidemics. A
person may bring some simple disease like measles into a community that has never been exposed to it before. The general
experience is that the virus hits very hard. Not only does it
spread like wildfire, but it tends to cause a more severe disease
in exposed susceptible adults than it does in the children who
form the susceptible group in our own communities. Thus, the
virus rampages for a while; it may cause some deaths, but
eventually it runs out of nonimmune hosts. If the community
is a remote one, there may not be another introduction of the
same virus for 20 or even 80 years. Even after that lapse of
time, the people who had been exposed the first time remain
immune. Only people born since the preceding epidemic contract the disease. The immunological memory function has been
so powerful and effective that people who had been exposed
once only, many decades previously, to the admittedly large
dose of the antigen involved in a frank infection rapidly eliminate the invader. It never gains a foothold in the tissues and
thus cannot cause disease.

The severity of virgin soil epidemics holds some salutary
lessons for us. There are now large-scale programs in America
and elsewhere to wipe out completely diseases such as measles.
It is most important to realize that once such vaccination programs have begun, they must be continued indefinitely. Let us
suppose that, after ten years, every American has either had
measles or been immunized against it. Let us suppose further
that after twenty years, health authorities became lax about the

situation, and vaccination programs gradually stopped. Then some traveler from a less developed country might fly in, carrying measles in his throat. The lucky virus would encounter millions of young adults that had been neither exposed nor vaccinated. The result would certainly be an epidemic of unparalleled magnitude and severity. The answer: alerted physicians, an educated community, and regular booster shots for all.

At the moment, smallpox eradication poses some of these public health problems. At the time of writing this book, we believe it is totally gone from the world never to return. Many countries have ceased or reduced their vaccination programs, and rightly so on balance of risks and benefits. But public health officials must maintain adequate stocks of vaccine for a good number of years yet, in case an unexpected pocket has persisted in some unknown place. With this caveat, eradication must be the eventual public health goal for all infectious agents for which no animal reservoir exists.

12

IMMUNOLOGICAL
TOLERANCE

THE NOBEL PRIZE is universally agreed to be the highest honor that a scientist can receive and perhaps the greatest accolade that man can bestow on man. There have been eight Nobel prizes awarded to immunologists. Some recipients we have already met: the intrepid von Behring, who discovered antitoxic immunity and whose work has saved thousands from diseases like diphtheria and tetanus; and the Russian genius Metchnikoff, who discovered phagocytosis and who became the first famous victim of the "brain drain" when he was persuaded to leave Russia and establish a laboratory at the Pasteur Institute in Paris. Another immunologist, the Austrian Karl Landsteiner, who discovered the human blood groups in 1901, went one step further than Metchnikoff. Despite 20 years of consistent achievement and his immense international reputation, Landsteiner was not paid enough in post-World War I Austria to support his family; he moved across the Atlantic to the Rockefeller Institute in New York in 1922. Only eight years later did the supreme recognition come. The award of the Nobel prize to G. M. Edelman and R. R. Porter in 1972 for their discovery of the structure of IgG was a fitting tribute to the immense importance that this understanding has had in elucidating nature's strategy for immune defenses.

The remaining three immunological Nobel laureates are linked in the most amazing way over half a century and half a globe through their profound interest in the subject matter of this chapter. Each in a way discovered immunological tolerance. The detailed story represents a fragment of modern history well worth recording.

Paul Ehrlich, the first of our trio, was the giant of German science in the early part of this century. He was a great chemist but was even more profoundly interested in biology. The microbial world and the host-parasite relationship fascinated him, and no aspect more so than the body's capacity to form antibodies. His dream was to combine chemistry and biology to devise rational treatments for infectious diseases. His idea was to construct "magic bullets" which would move in the bloodstream and exert a toxic action on microbes while leaving the host tissue cells unscathed. His discovery of arsenical drugs for the treatment of syphilis was a partial fulfillment. But again and again his thinking and writing would come back to the problem of antibodies and how the body formed them. He kept harking back to the idea of *Normalantikörper* (natural antibodies), which the system could make even before the antigen came along, and to the concept that active production implied simply a *Mehrleistung* (greater achievement) on the part of the antigenically stimulated system. In this respect he clashed sharply with Landsteiner, who insisted that antibody formation represented an *Andersleistung*, or chemically changed achievement, on the part of the body. This controversy raged for 50 years. In the context of the present chapter, Ehrlich raised a notable point. He coined the phrase "horror autotoxicus" to describe the disastrous turmoil which might result if the body started making antibodies to its own constituents. After all, the red cells and serum proteins of one species cause good antibody formation when injected into another species. Why, then, does a person not form antibodies to his own red cells? This worried Ehrlich and he wrote about the subject at great length, but did not resolve it satisfactorily.

We must now travel 40 years and 12,000 miles to Melbourne, Australia, to a laboratory just 10 yards from where these lines are being written. Sir Frank Macfarlane Burnet, distinguished Australian virologist, had come across two technical papers which slowly began to fit together in his mind, and, incidentally, paved the way for switching his research from a study of viruses to one of immunity. The first paper was one concerning a virus disease of mice called lymphocytic choriomeningitis, or LCM. This virus, when injected into adult, susceptible mice, causes a fairly mild meningitis. It was found that some strains of mice were insusceptible to it. Closer study revealed that these were mice which had been infected with the virus as very early embryos while in the mother's uterus. In these animals, the virus grew very extensively, particularly in lymphoid organs, but caused no disease whatever! Moreover, even when the mice grew up, they formed no anti-LCM antibodies, either to the virus in their own body or to vaccine injections of it. In fact, we now know that when this immunological stalemate is broken, as can happen late in life, the formation of antibodies to the virus can do much damage, owing to the injurious effects of chronically persisting antigen-antibody complexes.

The second observation was made by Dr. Ray Owen, a geneticist then at Madison, Wisconsin. It related to the blood groups of cattle twins. Many twin cattle are derived from two separate fertilized ova, and are thus nonidentical. They are neither more nor less closely related to each other than any two brothers or sisters. However, in contradistinction to man, the cattle share a common, single placenta, or afterbirth. In the placenta, extensive mingling of the blood of the two developing embryos occurs. This mixing includes large numbers of red cells as well as white cells and plasma. Accordingly, when the cattle are born, each contains some red cells made by itself, but also a large number of red cells which were made by the other twin. As the two twins were not identical, there was every chance that they would have different blood groups. In that case, one might expect that the young calf would soon form antibodies and reject its twin's red cells, which are, after all, good antigens. However, no such thing happened. The red cells, though genetically and antigenically foreign, lived on quite happily in their adopted host. No antibodies to them were formed.

Burnet, like Ehrlich 40 years earlier, was fascinated by the question of recognition in the immune system. How do the lymphocytes recognize "self" from "not-self"? How does the body dispose of unwanted, worn-out constituents arising within it (such as aging red cells) without an apparent immune response while dealing with foreign matter from the outside world largely through antibody formation? He felt that this problem of self-recognition was crucial to the whole understanding of antibody formation. The two studies just described gave him the key. In 1949 he and his colleague, Professor Frank Fenner, published a theoretical book which clearly predicted the discovery of tolerance. They formulated the view that if an antigen were introduced into an animal before the lymphoid system had matured, the developing animal would be tricked into recognizing the substance as "self." It would form no antibodies to it at the time, nor would it if injected with the same material in later life. The LCM virus and twin-cattle red-cell findings would then fit into place. In each case, the antigen had been present in the body from an early embryonic stage on. According to the theory, each would henceforth be handled as a "self" material, without antibody formation. The significance of this concept for a healthy body economy is obvious. The lymphoid system matures relatively late in embryonic development. Most of the potentially antigenic substances and certainly all the major constituents of the circulation are developed earlier in embryogenesis. Thus, according to the theory, the immature lymphoid system is already faced with these molecules from the moment of its first beginnings. The animal never gains the capacity to react to these materials. In fact, it would exhibit *immunological tolerance* to them.

The advantage of Burnet and Fenner's formulation was that it could be put to an experimental test. Burnet and his collaborators took fertile hen's eggs, and at various stages of incubation of the developing chick embryo, injected it with vaccine. If the theory was right, the chick would hatch and eventually grow up into an immunologically mature bird. It should be capable of forming perfectly adequate amounts of antibody to all antigens except the one used to vaccinate it in its embryonic life. To this antigen, it should fail to respond. The results of the experiment were distinctly anticlimactic. In fact, no modification of the host response was achieved! We now know the technical reasons for this failure, and will discuss them in detail. Sir Macfarlane Burnet still regards this experiment as one of the major disappointments in his distinguished career.

For the final chapter in our drama we must return to the Old World. In the early 1940s a young British zoologist, now Sir Peter Medawar, wanted to apply his interests in the skin to some problem related to the war effort. Fortunately, he came into association with a Scottish plastic surgeon, Mr. Thomas Gibson. Together they did experiments on grafting skin onto severely burned patients. Skin from a human donor healed onto the wound quite well, but within some days became red and angry looking, soon turned black, and dropped off altogether. If then slices of skin were taken from a different part of the patient's own body, it healed in and survived indefinitely. Medawar and Gibson soon came to embrace the hypothesis that an immunological process was at work in skin graft rejection. In a classical series of studies, Medawar proved the validity of this idea in experimental animals. He noted that skin graft rejection was due to the efforts of immunologically activated lymphocytes, and that a second graft from a given donor was rejected more rapidly and vigorously than the first, showing the existence of specific immunological memory.

In the early 1950s, Medawar and two colleagues, Drs. Rupert Billingham and Leslie Brent, became aware of Burnet and Fenner's little book on self-recognition. They also had given much thought to Owen's twin cattle, and Burnet's theory prompted a definitive test. The experiment, which they reported in 1953, is shown schematically on Figure 12–1. It employed different strains of inbred mice because it is possible to perform so many sequential brother-sister matings in mice that they soon become as similar to one another as identical twins. Let us consider two strains of mice that we designate A and B. All the A mice will accept skin grafts from other A mice because the intensive inbreeding has made them genetically identical. Similarly B mice will accept skin grafts from other B mice. However, if A skin is grafted onto B mice or vice versa, rapid rejection will follow. Medawar and his colleagues took inbred female A mice that had been mated to A males. When they were in the late stages of pregnancy, by a delicate operation, they injected living spleen cells from a B-strain donor animal. The mother was then left undisturbed to have her young. These were born and eventually grew up. As adults, they received a B-strain skin graft. This was indeed recognized as self. It took and thrived indefinitely. The mice were specifically incapable of reacting to the antigens of the B strain, although skin from a third strain, C, was promptly rejected. For the first time a state of immunological tolerance had been created in the laboratory.

Why did the skin graft experiment succeed where Burnet's inoculations had failed? We now know that this was chiefly because tolerance induction requires both an adequate dose and prolonged persistence of antigen in the tissues. One shot of a

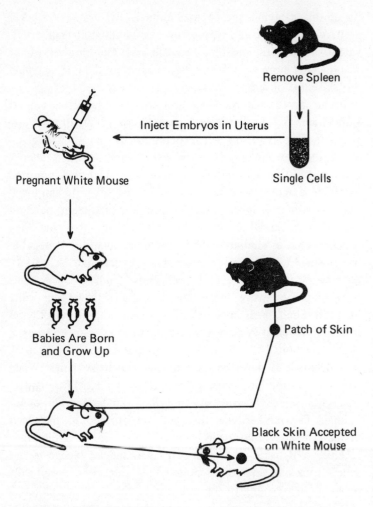

Figure 12–1. The induction of immunological tolerance to transplant antigens.

killed vaccine rarely achieves these twin aims. However, when living spleen cells are injected, they settle down in the host and proliferate, thus providing a continuing source of a considerable amount of antigen. The same two features of adequate dosage and persistence characterize the two natural examples of immunological tolerance—LCM infection in mice infected as tiny embryos, and acceptance of fraternal red cells in cattle twins.

For their separate contributions to the field of immunological tolerance, Burnet and Medawar shared the Nobel Prize for Physiology and Medicine in 1960. Many problems raised by their work still remain unsolved and are the subject of very active research. The chief scientists involved in this kind of work met in London in 1956 under the auspices of the Royal Society and a definition of immunological tolerance was accepted. Immunological tolerance represented a specific central failure of the immune response to an antigen engendered by exposing an animal to that antigen when its immune system was still immature.

Mechanisms of Immunological Tolerance

There is a natural desire to explain such a profound phenomenon as immunological tolerance by a single, unique mechanism. However, we have seen how delicate and manifold are the controls operating in the immune system, and in particular how many negative control or suppressor loops can operate. This being the case, it is evident that many of the experimental models used over the years in the study of tolerance highlight different mechanisms by which immunological nonreactivity can be obtained. Furthermore, given the large variety of concentrations, molecular forms, and tissue distribution patterns of self-antigens, it is evident that these, too, fail to elicit immune responses for a variety of reasons; that is, there are multiple mechanisms for self-tolerance.

There are four background concepts which must be mentioned before the mechanisms of tolerance are described. First, self-tolerance is not genetically built in to the immune system. It is acquired during the maturation of the system, separately in each individual of the species. This has been shown convincingly by an intriguing study. Recall the capacity of strain A mice to react vigorously to strain B tissues. It is possible to take a mouse embryo at a very early stage after fertilization, before it has implanted into the wall of the uterus, and place it into short-term tissue culture with another mouse embryo in such a way that the two little nests of cells fuse into one bigger nest. This can then be reimplanted into a foster-mother's uterus and amazingly, instead of giving rise to twins, *one* individual mouse results. This extraordinary creature thus has four parents, and is called a *tetraparental* or *allophenic* mouse. If one pair of parents of strain A was white, and the other pair of strain B black, the mouse would grow up not grey, but black-and-white-striped! The reason for this is that the individual cells of the tetraparental mouse do not fuse. They retain their A or B character. The mouse is simply a mixture of A and B cells, each cell exhibiting its own genetic characteristics. Such mice grow up perfectly healthy. There is no sign that they are reacting internally in any form of immunological civil war. Now, genetically, A mice are strong anti-B reactors and vice-versa. The mutual tolerance that the tetraparental's A lymphocytes display towards all B antigens, and vice versa, is thus clearly *somatically acquired*.

The second point is that tolerance is a quantitative rather than an absolute concept. Both in laboratory models of tolerance and in self-tolerance, the reduction in immune reactivity may not be absolutely to zero. A moment's consideration of some of the concepts we met in Chapter 5 gives the reason why. There is degeneracy and redundancy in the immune system, and thus a good deal of cross-reactivity among antigens. An antibody-combining site reactive to high affinity with a typhoid bacillus may, by chance, exhibit low affinity for an antigen on the animal's red cells. If all reactivities, of no matter how low an affinity, against all self-antigens were eliminated by the immune system, there would be a fair risk of wiping out the whole library of clonotypes. It suffices that, in a given operational setting, those clones of sufficiently high affinity to react significantly to the concentrations of self-antigens likely to be encountered are eliminated or functionally silenced. Thus, low-avidity B cell clones to some self-antigens can be found in the body. It is even possible to detect small amounts of low-avidity anti-self antibodies against some tissue antigens in the bloodstream. As long as various control mechanisms keep these at a low level, no harm results and there has even been speculation concerning possible useful roles of such antibodies.

The third point is that tolerance can be within the T cell and the B cell compartment, or, on occasion, within the T cell compartment alone. Under most circumstances, B cell triggering requires T cell help. Therefore, self-reactive B cells, even if present, could not get going in the absence of T cells reactive to some portion of the antigen concerned. Tolerance induction is obviously a concentration-dependent event: the higher the concentration of the tolerogen, the greater the degree of tolerance achieved, i.e., the more clones of relatively low avidity silenced. However, the concentration thresholds are different between T and B cells, T cells requiring lower concentrations of antigen than B cells. Therefore, for an antigen present in low concentration in the blood stream, such as the thyroid product thyroglobulin, there may be T cell tolerance but no B cell tolerance. This can spell trouble if a slight variant of the molecule is artificially introduced into the body, such as rabbit thyroglobulin into a mouse. T cells recognize any new determinant on the slightly different molecule, and help B cells to form antibodies to *all* the determinants, including those of the mouse's own thyroglobulin. An artificially induced autoimmune disease results.

Fourth, there are some self-antigens which never circulate at all, and which therefore do not reach the maturing lymphoid system and do not cause tolerance. Antigens on spermatozoa serve as an example. It is easy to cause autoantibody formation against them by artificial injections. Release of such sequestered antigens by viruses damaging the tissues can cause autoimmune disease.

Clonal Abortion

Of the various mechanisms responsible for tolerance, one termed clonal abortion is probably the most important. The concept is depicted in Figure 12–2. The reader will recall that mature virgin lymphocytes are made by an elaborate process

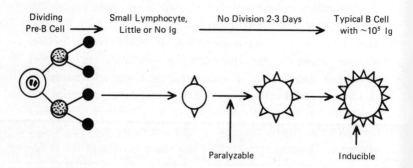

Figure 12–2.   B cell maturation in newborn spleen. The B cell emerges from the dividing cycles which generate it, possessing few or no surface Ig receptors. These are acquired in progressively larger amounts over the next two to three days. It is possible that the maturing cell with relatively few receptors is rapidly rendered tolerant on contact with antigen.

in the primary lymphoid organs. As a late stage in the process, they acquire their surface receptors for antigen. This does not happen all at one jump, but over a period of a couple of days. Clonal abortion implies that contact with the antigen with which that cell is capable of reacting will switch it off or perhaps even lead to its destruction. By such a mechanism, self-antigens would catch all the potentially self-reactive clones before they had matured into cells competent to mount an immune response, thereby nipping autoimmunity in the bud.

For the B cell, clonal abortion is an established fact for some antigens. It turns out that cells which have just acquired their IgM receptors, or some of them, can be switched off by antigen present in submicrogram concentrations per milliliter. In fact, an anti-immunoglobulin serum capable of uniting with Ig receptors on the surface of all new B cells, can act as a type of universal tolerogen. For example, fetal liver cells can be taken out of a mouse embryo before any B cells have developed. They can be placed in tissue culture, where, within a few days, B cells begin to appear. If, at the initiation of such cultures, some antiglobulin antibody is added to the cultures, the process of normal B cell maturation is aborted, and no B cells ever appear.

The mechanism of clonal abortion is under study, and one interesting finding has been noted in the antiglobulin model. If B cells are treated with antiglobulin, a characteristic series of movements of surface Ig molecules occurs (which will be described in detail in Chapter 13), the end result of which is a temporary disappearance of the surface Ig. In mature B cells, this is followed by a rapid reappearance of the receptors within six to eight hours. In newly born B cells with the IgM receptors just out, the early "disappearance trick" occurs but the receptors fail to be resynthesized. Such a "blind" lymphocyte, without receptors, obviously cannot "see" antigen and cannot react to it. This irreversible disappearance may be occurring in reactions to self-antigens when they hit immature B cells. If so, the result would be specific tolerance.

It is probable that clonal abortion occurs for T cells as well, though the mechanisms have not been investigated because the T cell receptors are so much harder to study. It is certain that the end result of the induction of tolerance to skin graft (histocompatibility) antigens is an absence of clones of cells capable of recognizing those antigens.

Extension of the Concept of Tolerance to Adult Animals

Before describing the other known mechanisms of tolerance induction, it is important to note that circumstances exist for inducing tolerance also when adult animals are injected with antigens. Two chief forms, with variants, exist. The first is when an antigen *itself not capable of causing immunity* is given in sufficient dose and over a sufficient period of time. A good example is that of a foreign serum protein, such as human IgG injected into a mouse. If great care is taken to remove all aggregates from the preparation, it fails to cause antibody formation, probably because it does not get onto macrophage surfaces. If the dose given is sufficiently high, tolerance is noted within a few days. The second example is when a large (supraimmunogenic) dose of some highly polymeric antigens is given to an adult animal. This kind of nonreactivity was first noted with a polysaccharide from pneumococci about 40 years ago, and the term immunological paralysis was used to describe it.

Explanations for Tolerance and Paralysis of Adult Animals

Several explanations offer themselves for the above findings. First, suppressor T cells certainly account for a proportion of the results. They have been strongly implicated in many of the experimental models where tolerance is induced by a multiplicity of injections, and in some but not all of the experiments using bland, disaggregated antigens or highly polymeric antigens. Second, a simple blockade of receptors is involved in some cases. We discussed in Chapter 9 the fact that not every encounter between a cell receptor and an antigen need trigger. If receptors on a lymphocyte are occupied by nonimmunogenic antigen, then that lymphocyte will be impeded from reacting with a depot of potentially immunogenic antigen as on a macrophage surface. Third, there is evidence that excessive concentrations of some highly polymeric antigens can cause the irreversible receptor disappearing trick even in mature B cells, similar to that so commonly seen in immature B cells.

There is one variant of the polymeric antigen story of great practical interest. We saw in Chapter 3 how antibodies can cause antigen molecules to become aggregated. It turns out that soluble complexes formed in the zone of slight antigen excess (ones in which there are still antigenic determinants free to react with lymphocyte receptors) represent antigens powerfully capable of paralyzing both T and B cells. The mechanism may involve receptor blockade or disappearance. The practical importance of this is that it constitutes a way of lowering immune responses specifically when large amounts of antigen coexist in the body with substantial amounts of antibody. Such is the case for cancer antigens in late cancer. The complexes can also interfere with the function of immunocyte effector cells at both T and B cell level.

Does this multiplicity of ways of achieving tolerance or paralysis in the adult not pose some dangers, for example, in overwhelming infections? In most natural situations, a large-scale shutdown of immune defenses does not occur. For one thing, the early development of antibodies, even if not successful in getting rid of the microbe altogether, still ensures its removal from the circulation, and thus reduces its chances of meeting lymphocytes. For another, particulate antigens such as living microbes are usually immunogenic rather than tolerogenic. Finally, except for the case of suppressor cells (which represent an activation event and therefore really an immune response), tolerance involves antigens reaching all or most of the lymphocytes with a given reactivity. To achieve a significant reduction in immune potential, the microbes concerned (or large amounts of products from them) would have to penetrate into every nook and cranny of the lymphoid system. This is in contrast to an immune response, where only one lymphocyte can initiate clonal proliferation. In the adult animal suffering from infection, nature has clearly tipped the balance in favor of immunity. Nevertheless, failure of the immune response is a feature of advanced stages of several diseases, notably tuberculosis, leprosy, and cancer. Paralysis mechanisms could well play a role here.

Our knowledge of "self-recognition" has come a considerable distance since Paul Ehrlich coined his pithy phrase "horror autotoxicus." The question raises the most fundamental issues, not only about lymphocytes and antibodies, but about the nature of cellular interactions generally and the maintenance of bodily and tissue integrity. This chapter is designed to do no more than whet your appetite for a field which is advancing steadily and stands in the very forefront of research in many fields, including organ transplantation, autoimmunity, and cancer research.

13

IMMUNOCYTES AS MODEL CELLS

SCIENTISTS, as well as having to be good thinkers, are also great pragmatists. They realize when a new technique or a new idea opens up a field for extensive experimentation. They then crowd to it like bees searching for honey, each bringing the background and perspectives of different past experiences. This swarming behavior of scientists not only makes narrow research fields able to move very quickly, but also ensures a good deal of cross-fertilization. The new idea or technique is the focal point; the wide diversity of skills and orientations of the scientists attracted to it is a force for generalization, for spread. In this respect, the boom in immunology can be said to be a good thing not only for immunologists but for science as a whole. Certainly, its central tenets are widely known and its key techniques of value in a myriad of studies that have nothing to do with immunology per se. In fact, we see two phenomena here. On the one hand, scientists from backgrounds as far apart as biochemistry and vascular surgery come to study some specialized aspect of immunology of interest to them, and thereby add to immunology itself. On the other, an immunological creature, such as a lymphocyte or an antibody molecule tagged with a fluorescent dye, may serve as a model for some purpose that

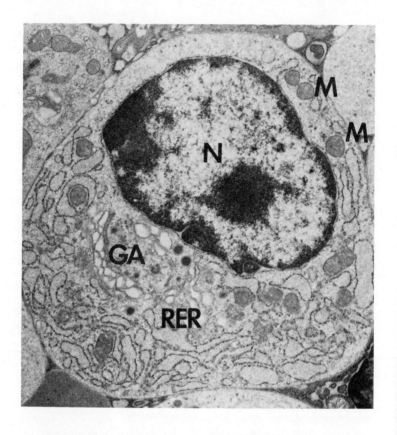

Figure 13–1.　Chief electron-micrographic features of a plasma cell.

N　　　　nucleus
M　　　　mitochondria
GA　　　Golgi apparatus
RER　　　rough-surfaced endoplasmic reticulum

is not quintessentially immunological at all, thereby making immunology generally the servant of biology.

In this chapter, I have selected two examples of immunocytes acting as model cells. They have been chosen as representing phenomena of central importance both within immunology and transcending it. One is rather old, the other rather new.We shall begin with the former.

Plasma Cells and Their Properties

In Chapters 4 and 5, we discussed briefly the fascinating subject of differentiation, the process by which unspecialized and rapidly dividing cells gave rise to progeny with increasingly sophisticated skills. We must note something that applies also to certain extremely gifted human beings. The super-specialist, the prodigy, the single-minded expert will frequently be so dedicated to the task at hand that he will be relatively hopeless in any sphere of human achievement other than his own specialty. The plasma cell, which we here put under the microscope, is a prodigy of specialization. It is a cell type created for one purpose only—the synthesis of a given antibody. This one task it performs to perfection, and, as far as we can tell, a plasma cell has no other useful function. By learning about it, we will incidentally learn much about the biochemistry of cells in general.

Structure of Plasma Cells as Revealed by Electron Microscopy

A diagram of a plasma cell as it appears under the electron microscope is shown in Figure 13–1. By far the most prominent and characteristic feature of the cell is an elaborate series of stacks of double membranes which fill practically the whole of the cytoplasm. Each double membrane is separated from the next by a sac which contains almost pure antibody. Each membrane is studded with a row of closely spaced dark-staining dots which represent structures called ribosomes. The technical name for this ribosome-rich membrane system is rough-surfaced endoplasmic reticulum. So extensive and space-filling is this reticulum that the nucleus is pushed right to one side of the cell. This eccentrically placed, relatively small nucleus in a cell with bulky cytoplasm is a characteristic feature of plasma cells, also readily recognized under the light microscope.

Plasma cells also possess a second type of internal membrane system consisting of multiple-layered stacks of membrane flanked by a large number of tiny droplet-like bags or vesicles. This structure sits just next to the nucleus. In the light microscope it shows up as a zone of pale-staining cytoplasm. This is termed the Golgi complex of the cell.

The final feature of the plasma cell is that it contains moderately large numbers of ovoid organelles termed mitochondria. These are very characteristic and easily spotted because they contain numerous ridges which appear to grow inward from their walls.

Let us now see what is the function of each of these portions of the cell. The nucleus is the brain center of the cell. It possesses the DNA which contains the coded instructions or blueprints for the manufacture of any material that the cell can make. Among a myriad of other things, it contains blueprints for antibody manufacture. The specifications for the synthesis of both light and heavy immunoglobulin chains are encoded in the sequence of the four subunits of DNA which go to make up the long, polymerized DNA molecule. You would not think that four letters could code for anything very elaborate. The way that nature has managed this is by joining the four letters up into sets of triplets. With the basic building blocks of DNA (adenine, thymine, guanine, and cytosine, or A, T, G, and C for short) we can construct 64 three-letter words. Each of these triplets is a code word corresponding to an amino acid. As there are only 20 amino acids, and not 64, there is information to spare. In fact, quite a number of amino acids are coded for by several different triplets.

Coded instructions are not much good if they can't be sent anywhere. We have said that the DNA must remain stably in its place in the nucleus of the cell. One of the chief functions of the nucleus is the manufacture of a coded copy of the DNA instructions. This is in the form of another kind of nucleic acid called ribonucleic acid or RNA. There are several kinds of RNA. The variety which carries the coded instructions for the amino-acid sequence of a protein from the gene in the nucleus to the synthetic factory in the cytoplasm is appropriately named messenger RNA.

The messenger RNA leaves the nucleus and travels to the cytoplasm. Now it comes into association with the little dots called ribosomes. The ribosomes can "read" the RNA message in somewhat the same way that the output device of a business machine can read punched paper tape. Ribosomes actually travel along the strand of messenger RNA and, as decoding proceeds, enzymes hook together the growing polypeptide chain. Naturally, the length of the protein synthesized will depend on the length of the messenger strand. For every three RNA letters (nucleotides) there will be one amino acid. Moreover, it is efficient that more than one ribosome should be reading the message at one time. In fact, usually a series of ribosomes attaches itself to a messenger RNA strand and the spacing between individual ribosomes is relatively even—around 90 or so nucleotide units. In other words, if a messenger RNA strand codes for an immunoglobulin light chain, which is 214 amino acids long, it will itself require 642 nucleotide units to do the coding. In fact, the light-chain messenger is considerably larger than that, because there are important structural bits of it which have no coding function but are needed to give the messenger the right shape for attachment to the ribosome. Every messenger RNA contains a long string of poly-A, which has been useful in its isolation for study. This noncoding portion aside, a further complexity arises from the fact that proteins are first synthesized somewhat longer than their final form. A portion that is needed for movement from ribosomes through the membrane of the endoplasmic reticulum is clipped off by a "clippase" enzyme even before the chain is completed. Other pieces of microsurgery may also be performed on proteins before they leave the cell in their final form. These considerations aside, the length of the messenger RNA determines how many ribosomes attach to it. For the Ig light-chain messenger RNA seven ribosomes fit on, and as they travel along the strand, seven light chains will be formed simultaneously. The whole structure of messenger RNA and associated ribosomes is called a polysome.

In mammalian cells, the same messenger tape can be played over and over again. As a ribosome comes to the end of a messenger tape, one completed protein chain is released. The ribosome can then reatttach itself to the beginning of the messenger RNA and the whole process starts again. In long-lived plasma cells, the indication is that messenger RNA molecules are very stable and can be "read" a great number of times.

In the plasma cell, as well as in other secretory cells such as the pancreas, which has been extensively studied, the polysomes are attached to the double membranes of the rough-surfaced endoplasmic reticulum. Newly formed proteins are jetted across into the space between two apposed membranes. The light and heavy chains are made on two separate sets of polysomes (seven ribosomes per light-chain polysome and about 15 per heavy-chain polysome). Assembly into full Ig molecules takes place by mechanisms that are not yet well understood. The first few sugars of the carbohydrate side chains of Ig are added to the molecule in the endoplasmic reticulum. The molecules gradually move through the spaces of the endoplasmic reticulum towards the portion which is nearest the Golgi apparatus. Then, tiny smooth-surfaced vesicles containing antibody bud off from the endoplasmic reticulum by a process akin to that seen in Figure 6–1. They move towards the Golgi complex and fuse with what is termed its "forming" face. The Golgi complex consists of an interconnected series of membrane-bound stacks serving as a concentrating and packaging center. Within it, the terminal sugars are added to glycoproteins, both those destined for secretion and those which will become membrane receptors. Finally, membrane-bound vesicles bud off from the "maturing" face of the Golgi complex, containing the protein for export. These tiny secretory vesicles make their way to the cell surface, where they fuse with the cell membrane and discharge their contents by the exact reverse of the process of phagocytosis (Figure 6–1).

You will note that extreme compartmentation is part of nature's design. In fact, the immunoglobulin had to cross a membrane only once, that is, during its travel from the ribosome across the endoplasmic reticulum; and an elaborate, specialized machinery is known to exist for that. During all the rest of its sojourn in the cell, it remained behind membrane barriers of various sorts, sequestered from the cell sap or cytosol.

The orderly process of intracellular transport and secretion can continue even if protein synthesis is stopped by specific inhibitors. However, transport does require energy, as indeed do many of the reactions occurring inside cells. This is where the mitochondria come in. These are the powerhouses of the cell. Their chief job is to convert the energy released by the burning of the cell's foodstuffs into a form that is generally useful for the myriad energy-consuming chemical reactions which take place in any cell. The energy is stored in the form of energy-rich phosphate bonds in molecules of a substance called adenosine triphosphate, or ATP. When this molecule is converted to adenosine diphosphate or ADP, free energy is released, which can drive all kinds of synthetic processes. Mitochondrial action ensures that a good level of ATP is maintained in the cell. All animal cells contain some mitochondria, and plasma cells contain rather more than average.

While electron microscopic study gives us the most complete picture of plasma cell structure, a good deal of knowledge about plasma cells can also be obtained through the light microscope. Three features stand out: the eccentric nucleus, the prominent Golgi zone, and the bulky cytoplasm rich in nucleic acids. When sections of lymph nodes are stained with dyes that have special affinity for RNA, the plasma cells take up the color because of their high RNA content and stain brilliantly. This allows them to be spotted even at quite low magnifications.

It is frequently stated that cell division and specialized cell function are antithetical and mutually exclusive events. The extreme example cited is the brain cell, which performs a highly specialized task and never divides. In antibody formation, however, division and specialized function overlap to a significant extent. It is true that the plasmablast ancestors of plasma cells synthesize less antibody than do their final offspring. However, these rapidly dividing cells are already sufficiently sophisticated to form some antibody. In fact, the oversimplified view should be modified. As a broad generalization it is true to say that rapidly dividing cells are more likely to retain a multiplicity of potential and less likely to be restricting their activities to one major task than are nondividing cells. However, antibody formation is only one of many examples in biology in which the gradual emergence of full commitment to a given task can be noted.

One Cell, One Antibody

The specialization of plasma cells is far more subtle and more profound than has been realized thus far. In fact, not only is the plasma cell specialized for antibody formation in general, but each plasma cell can manufacture only one particular and unique chemical type of antibody.

This property can be illustrated by immunizing an animal with four antigens, A, B, C, and D. These are all taken up in lymph nodes and spleen, and often one macrophage may contain all four antigens. Within a few days, the lymphatic tissues will be churning out considerable quantities of anti-A, anti-B, anti-C, and anti-D antibodies. One can then kill the animal, prepare a white-cell suspension from the lymph node, isolate individual plasma cells, incubate them singly in microdroplets, and then test each droplet for its content of each of the four antibodies. The result is that some cells form anti-A, some anti-B, some anti-C, and some anti-D antibodies. Each cell forms only one antibody. Each cell is considerably more restricted in its synthetic potential than the lymph node or spleen as a whole.

In Chapter 3, we discussed how one antigen could call forth antibodies of five different chemical and genetic classes. It turns out that, with rare exceptions, each plasma cell can make only one class of antibody at one time. In the above example, the population of anti-A forming cells can be further broken down into subpopulations: some cells form anti-A IgG, some anti-A

IgM, and so forth. Although, locked within its nucleus, each cell has the blueprints for the synthesis of the other immunoglobulin classes, some genetic switching mechanism restricts active antibody formation to only one class. The rest of the cell's genetic reserve remains irrevocably sealed away inside the nucleus.

Plaque Method for Studying Antibody-Forming Cells

While micromanipulation methods gave us a good deal of information about plasma cells, their great disadvantage is their tediousness, which limits the number of cells that can be studied. A vital methodological breakthrough was made by Dr. Niels K. Jerne and his collaborators Claudia Henry and Albert Nordin in 1963, when they discovered a technique whereby single antibody-forming cells could be detected, enumerated, and studied by a simple, reliable, and rapid method. The method, called the hemolytic plaque technique, is shown in Figure 13–2. Let us illustrate its virtues by describing Jerne's original experiment.

Animals, such as mice, are given an injection of the antigen, sheep red blood cells, directly into a vein. Much of the antigen is captured by the spleen, and soon the lymphocytes in the spleen become induced into antibody formation. If one has injected a series of mice at one time, one can kill individual mice at sequential time points after the antigenic stimulus. The spleen is then removed, chopped into fine pieces with scissors, and forced through a fine wire mesh. The mechanical stresses break up the fabric of the spleen, which essentially falls apart into its component single cells. These can then be suspended in a tissue-culture medium. Next, the suspension of mouse spleen cells (which may contain a small proportion of antibody-formers) is mixed with a suspension of sheep red blood cells

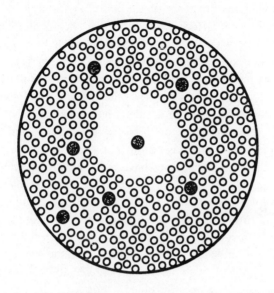

Figure 13–2. The hemolytic plaque method for the detection of single antibody-forming cells.

in a ratio of about 100 sheep red cells for every mouse white cell. A layer of the mixture is then poured into a glass container. Stable spatial relationships between the mouse white cells and the sheep red cells are preserved, either by incorporating a jellifying agent into the suspension, or by ensuring a very thin, even layer of fluid and cells in specially constructed glass chambers. The preparations are next heated to 37°C (blood heat) and incubated for half an hour. This is sufficient time for an antibody-synthesizing cell to secrete the antibody into the medium in the immediate vicinity. This is avidly soaked up by the sheep red cells (remember the antigen which originally stimulated the mice *was* sheep red cells). If a small amount of the serum factor called "complement" is added, the antibody-soaked sheep red cells will rapidly burst and disappear. This results in a circular zone of clearing or "lysis" in the immediate surrounds of the antibody-forming cells. Such an area of lysis is technically termed a "hemolytic plaque." It can be seen with the naked eye, but much more accurately with a low-power microscope. It is a matter of great ease to count the number of hemolytic plaques which one whole spleen is capable of giving rise to—in other words, to enumerate the antibody-forming cells in a spleen at a given stage of the immune response. Studies of this sort have shown that the true latent period for antibody production is less than a day. In general, such plaque techniques have much greater sensitivity than does an examination of the serum for antibody content.

It is not necessary to use red blood cells as the antigen. Many proteins, carbohydrates, or haptens have been used, and the antigen is then artificially coated onto the sheep red blood cells for the revelation step. This plaque technique has revolutionized immunology with its sensitivity, versatility, and applicability to a wide range of problems. For example, we owe to it the discovery of both helper and suppressor T cells. Further, virtually all the observations that have been made through lymphocytes making antibodies in tissue culture are "read out" by plaque techniques.

The Fluid Mosaic Model of the Cell Membrane

We turn now to a second, newer, and essentially less immunological subject area extensively fertilized by the humble lymphocyte. It is the current concept of the cell membrane, the vital skin of each cell that separates it from its neighbors and from the extracellular fluids.

Until a decade ago, this subject was of rather specialized interest, but it has exploded at a rate perhaps even faster than that of immunology. Why? First, because a new unifying hypothesis has made it universally accessible. Second, because of the excitement about allosteric changes, cyclic nucleotides, and the internal message system of the cell that were discussed in Chapter 9. Third, because membranes are intimately involved in the discourse between cells, and thus in problems like transmission of impulses in the nervous system, and differentiation of primitive cells into organs and tisues. Membranes, like the genetic code, represent another example of generalism in biology, another fundamental area of interest to all biologists.

Consider for a moment what the cell membrane must do. Obviously, it has to be a mechanical barrier stopping cell contents from flowing out, but equally obviously, it must not be rigidly impermeable so as to allow inflow of nutrients. The permeability must be *selective*, that is, kidney cells must "know" to let some molecules pass into the urine and to retard others, while the permeability characteristics of placenta cells or stomach-lining cells will be quite different. Furthermore, the cell membrane must be *reactive*. Impulses and stimuli are reaching it all the time—hormones, nutrients, chemical transmitter substances which resemble drugs, serum proteins, and, of course, physical contacts with other cells. The membrane must be constructed to ensure that each cell responds appropriately to the signals reaching it. Finally, the cell membrane must be *dynamic*. It must move and even propel the cell, in the case of motile cells; it must grow and split in the case of dividing cells; it must maintain its integrity during processes of ingestion or secretion of materials; it must allow for the replenishment of receptor molecules that are shed off during the cell's life. All of these requirements show the need for an information function of sophisticated nature as well as the requisite physical structure.

While our discussion here will be limited to the skin of the cell, the so-called plasma membrane, we should note that there are also numerous, very clever internal membranes, such as those of the mitochondria, where enzymes for energy production must be lined up in complex arrays; and the curious double

membrane layer surrounding the nucleus of the cell and sep-
arating it from the cytoplasm.

How did nature solve the problem of the cell membrane? A
schematic and partial answer is given in Figure 13–3. Much of
the mechanical barrier function and the dynamic properties are
provided by a so-called lipid bilayer which is cunningly designed.
There is a double layer of fatty molecules consisting of fatty
acid side chains and phosphate-containing areas called polar
head groups. The double layer is arranged so that the fatty
"tails" face each other, while the polar "heads" face away from

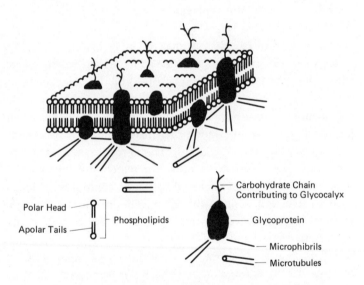

Figure 13–3. Schematic view of the cell membrane. Protein molecules, with or without attached carbohydrates, are
seen as floating in a sea of phospholipids. Some proteins
span the membrane, others are embedded in either the
outer or the inner leaf. Some proteins may be tethered by
microfibrils. Microtubules are frequently found just inside
the membrane, but their exact relationship to membrane
proteins and microfibrils remains uncertain.

each other. The fatty portions repel water; they are hydrophobic. Thus, water and molecules dissolved in water do not want to enter. As this comprises most of the molecules in a cell, an effective barrier is created. The polar head groups are water-loving, or hydrophilic. They make friends happily with the inner cytoplasm and the outer extracellular fluid. This helps a natural orientation of the fatty acids and stops flip-flop movements that could threaten the membrane's integrity. The fatty molecules are not static; they move and flow and spin at a rapid rate, but they invert only very rarely. The phospholipids immediately in contact with membrane proteins move less freely and influence the protein's shape.

The informational function of the membrane is contained in the proteins of the membrane. Each type of cell has its characteristic set of proteins. These float, as single molecules or small combinations of molecules, like little icebergs in the sea of fat. The membrane is in fact a mosaic of proteins and lipids in a fluid and highly dynamic state. The proteins can interact with each other or can meet and be buckled by other substances that reach them. Some of the proteins span the membrane completely with bits sticking out into the extracellular milieu and other bits into the watery inside of the cell. Other proteins sit mainly within one of the two bilayers, with a portion reaching to the inside or the outside, but not both. In every case, the molecules possess hydrophilic regions which interface with the watery milieu and hydrophobic, lipophilic portions that fit happily amidst the fats. The proteins are vectorially inserted into the membrane. There is no mistaking the inner and outer halves.

Many cells of the body exhibit polarity. For example, cells may have a base facing one way and hairy extensions called cilia another way. How is polarity consistent with the fluid mosaic model? Obviously, restrictions to movement of membrane proteins exist in such cells. One known restriction is imposed by *tight junctions* that cells make with other cells. Tight junctions are known to be capable of stopping the movement of certain enzymes across them.

Just inside the cell membrane, electron micrographs have shown us very fine fibrils that go right to the membrane itself. These microfibrils are thought to represent a kind of tethering mechanism for some of the transmembrane proteins, connecting with the microtubules which the electron microscope can see deeper in the cytoplasm. The microfibril mechanism is intimately involved in cell motility, and contains muscle-like contractile proteins. It is believed that these inner membrane proteins form a network-like cytoskeleton for the cell.

Just outside the membrane, certain electron-microscopic stains show the so-called glycocalyx. This is mainly carbohydrate in nature. Many of the important membrane proteins which have receptor functions possess chains of sugars attached to them; they are in fact *glycoproteins*, and the glycocalyx consists mainly of the carbohydrate chains of these molecules. The glycocalyx is important for cell-to-cell contact and cell migration.

Lymphocytes and the Plasma Membrane

The lymphocyte has many virtues for students of cell membranes. First, it is a cell that likes to lead a relatively independent existence and is not connected by physical bridges to other cells, as happens in most organized tissues. For this reason, lymphatic organs fall apart easily under mild mechanical stresses and yield single-cell suspensions with few damaged cells. Second, the protein receptors of the lymphocyte have been extensively studied, and a wide variety of important reagents and methods have been accumulated by immunologists. These are now available to the cell biologist for his purposes.

Third, an extraordinary phenomenon, now known to be much more general, was first discovered in lymphocytes, which we must now describe.

Capping the Lymphocyte

The fluidity of the membrane, and the free mobility of proteins within the plane of the membrane are well demonstrated by observing a process that has come to be called capping the lymphocyte. Consider the immunoglobulin receptors on mouse B lymphocytes. If one prepares in a rabbit an antiserum against mouse IgM, and then conjugates to this a fluorescent dye such as fluorescein or rhodamine, one can observe under the oil-immersion high-power lens of the ordinary microscope what happens to the IgM receptors when lymphocytes are exposed to anti-IgM. This is best done at 37°C. The process is summarized in Figure 13–4. First, within a matter of seconds, the completely smooth, uniformly distributed staining indicative of the random dispersion of the receptors on the B cell surface begins to be disrupted. Tiny spots, which may be likened to the first little granules appearing when milk sours, can be seen on the lymphocyte surface. Within minutes, these enlarge to become progressively bigger blobs of fluorescence on the cell surface. These can grow up to 0.5 microns in diameter. Simultaneously with the enlargement of fluorescent blobs, caused by the coalescence of the smaller spots, a second phenomenon can be noted, discernible within three minutes but reaching its height within five to fifteen minutes. It is the progressive movement of the blobs of fluorescence to one pole of the cell. At the completion of this process, the fluorescence picture resembles a beautiful crescent moon, all the receptors having moved to a cap covering a quarter to a half of the circumference of the cell profile. Fur-

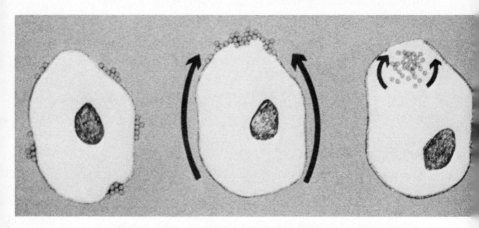

Figure 13–4. Patching and capping of lymphocyte receptors. When antibodies to a freely mobile cell membrane protein are added to a lymphocyte suspension, the individual protein molecules readily aggregate into patches by a process similar to the lattice formation described in Figure 3–4. These patches form even in a metabolically inactive cell. If the cell is healthy and at body temperature, the patches are swept into a "cap" at one pole of the cell and then the aggregated material is swallowed by the process described in Figure 6–1.

ther investigation shows that the patching is independent of cell metabolism—it occurs even when cells have been poisoned and is a purely physicochemical process. Capping, however, requires cell metabolism. If the fats of the cell membrane are turned into a lard-like state by cooling the cells down to 4°, patching as well as capping is prevented. The viscosity of the fatty "sea" is just too high to let the protein "icebergs" move freely.

Why does the anti-IgM cause these dramatic things to happen to the IgM receptors? The key to patching has been given already in Chapter 3. Patch formation is really rather like a precipitin reaction, occurring not in a test tube but in a two-dimensional plane. The anti-IgM itself is an IgG molecule, namely a bivalent antibody, with two combining sites per IgG molecule. The IgM receptor, consisting of two light chains and two heavy chains, is also bivalent with respect to any given one of its many anti-genic determinants. Cross-linking and lattice formation can occur and progress rapidly at 37°, as the cell's lipids are molten at this temperature.

The capping is not quite so easily explained. Apparently linking external molecules onto the receptors is a stimulus to lymphocyte mobility, and as the cell moves in one direction the heavy blobs tend to lag behind and get dragged into a trailing cap. This is not a full explanation, however, as there are circumstances where nonmotile cells can cap. While much about capping remains mysterious, we do know that specific poisons of microtubules (which are involved in cell mobility) inhibit the process.

Patching and capping can be induced in all B lymphocytes by antiglobulin, but a multivalent antigen can cap receptors of only those B lymphocytes specific for it. If populations of such lymphocytes are first prepared in a pure form, then a sequence of events identical to that induced with the model probe can be seen using fluorescent antigen.

The caps do not last long on the lymphocyte surface. A proportion of the receptor-antibody complexes is shed off, but the majority is simply swallowed by pinocytosis—a process very similar to phagocytosis (see Figure 6–1). Following the ingestion of the receptor-anti-receptor mixture, this is digested by the lysosomal mechanism and the bits are spat out by the cell. This process commences about 10 minutes after initiation of patching, is in full swing by 30 to 60 minutes, and is completed by two hours. This leaves the cell bereft of receptors. Normal, mature B cells then rapidly set about replacing their receptor coat. Within six to eight hours, the IgM is back. In the case of immature, "pre-B" cells this does not happen, and we discussed in Chapter 12 how important this is with respect to self-recognition.

What has particularly excited the imagination of both immunologists and cell biologists about this phenomenon of patching and capping is its possible physiological significance. The sequence is not unique for surface Ig receptors. Capping has been noted for many cell surface macromolecules including histocompatibility antigens and various cell differentiation markers. Moreover, it is not just antibodies which initiate the capping. True antigens and multivalent plant lectins can also be used. An obvious question to ask is whether the process may be involved in triggering cells. A very recent study on a different kind of cell, the mast cell, has suggested that the simple cross-linking of two surface receptors, without the formation of an actual lattice, can initiate its activation. It might well be that the coming together of two molecules tweaks their shape sufficiently to initiate an allosteric change and an enzymic chain reaction. Alternatively, the two molecules coming together may create a pore for calcium ions, which might do the triggering. Obviously, the free mobility of receptors and other proteins in the cell membrane opens up many possibilities for control mechanisms, such as the formation and dispersion of pores, the assembly of supramolecular aggregates or arrays of enzymes, the appropriate arrangement of junctions with other cells, and so forth. In many ways, the fluid mosaic model of the cell membrane has transformed our thinking.

Clearly this chapter has given only a few superficial examples from the broad fields of cell and molecular biology. As it is being written, the lay press is full of the news of the synthetic manufacture by a team at the Massachusetts Institute of Technology of a whole gene, not only its coding portion but complete with all the controls. The debate about genetic engineering and the desirability of continuing research on recombinant DNA rages on. These are among many signs that the great movement of modern biology is starting to be of concern to the layman. The dialogue between an increasingly informed society and the scientific community can only be of benefit to both.

14

GENETICS OF
TISSUE COMPATIBILITY

MOST PEOPLE share a sense of wonder when they see identical twins. There is something almost eerie about two human beings so alike that even close friends have difficulty telling them apart. Occasional sets of identical twins in a community are quaint and charming, but if the whole human race were composed of people that all looked exactly alike, much of the savor would go out of life. While no resemblance between people is quite as close as that between two identical twins, we readily recognize family likenesses. A little more remote, but nonetheless real, is the resemblance between people of a given national origin. Swedes do look different from Italians or from Irishmen. Yet all these Europeans resemble each other closely enough that we can group them together and differentiate them from, say, Asians. And, though at times some of one's friends make you wonder, it is not too difficult to tell a human from an ape. It takes no great amount of education to know all these things, but, believe it or not, the above paragraph was a brief lesson in genetics.

Genetic Mechanisms of Identity and Diversity

Genetics is a study of the genes of an organism, and it embraces all aspects of the way in which heredity works. The two identical twins are so alike because each started off with identical packages of DNA in the nucleus of the cell which finally grew into two persons. The DNA composition of a person is determined when one sperm cell from the father penetrates one egg cell or ovum from the mother. The nuclei of the sperm and the ovum fuse, and this fused cell divides a large number of times to give one individual. In the case of identical twins, an accident of nature occurs after the first cleavage of the fertilized egg, so that each of these two cells gives rise to one complete individual. Why are identical twins so much more alike than ordinary brothers and sisters? It is true that two individuals who have the same mother and father will have many similarities in their DNA. However, nature has devised a very effective mechanism to ensure that no two sperms or eggs from a given person are exactly alike. During the formation of the sperms, there is a complex scrambling mechanism which results in each sperm getting a somewhat different "mix" of a person's father's and mother's characteristics. The same is true of the egg. So, the sexual process engenders tremendous diversity. This is a far more powerful and rapid way of making sure that the whole human race is not composed of identical people than simply relying on mutation. Asexual life forms have only limited methods for genetic variation during their division. All those higher forms of life that replicate by sexual means have the extra mechanism of scrambling the components of the two parents. This sexual creation of diversity must be considered a major force in evolution, constantly allowing new forms to emerge and to be selected for survival.

This tendency for creation of diversity can be combated by

selective breeding. If a breeder of dogs wants to create a special strain of miniature dogs, he must first of all choose two small dogs of the opposite sex, mate them, and keep selecting the smallest of the progeny for mating. If he wishes to make sure that the progeny are not only small but also alike in other characteristics such as hair length, coat color, and length of tail, his quickest way is to embark on brother-sister mating. In experimental mice, it has been observed that about twenty successive generations in which only brothers and sisters are mated suffice to produce littermates that are so like each other that they will accept skin grafts mutually exchanged between them. All the littermates are as close to each other as identical twins. In fact, after such intensive inbreeding, one can now commence to mate the offspring of the inbred strain randomly. It will take about eight generations of such random matings before sufficient mutations build up to generate significant diversity. In this manner, very large stocks of inbred mice can be produced, and these are widely used in transplantation research. It will be obvious that this is not nature's way of arranging things. Animals in the field do not inbreed, and even the most primitive races of man have strong taboos against brother-sister marriages. Apart from the evolutionary advantages of diversity, inbreeding has the disadvantage of frequently bringing to light deleterious "recessive" genes that do no harm to an individual if he inherits the trait from only one of his parents, but seriously weaken him if he inherits it from both sides.

Application of Genetics to Transplantation

How do all the above considerations apply to transplantation? Genes dictate protein structure. Many proteins appear on the surface of the cell. Others are enzymes which may indirectly alter the surface of a cell. Therefore, if two individuals are different genetically, there will be surface differences between their cells. If cells from one individual are injected or grafted into another, the lymphoid system recognizes the surface differences. The foreign cells behave as *antigens*. Just as there are degrees of dissimilarity in appearance between people or dogs, so there are variations in the strength of disparity between the cell antigens. In other words, some cells will engender a more vigorous rejection response than others. To analyze these quantitative differences, we must now introduce some new terms.

A gene is a unit of inheritance defining a particular, identifiable characteristic. Under ideal circumstances, the gene product is a polypeptide chain of defined amino-acid sequence corresponding to a defined sequence of nucleotide triplets in the DNA of the gene. Frequently the geneticist has to settle for something less precise. He may find that some trait, such as eye color, or ability to taste a particular chemical, or tendency to form an unusual type of red blood cell, is inherited as a single unit. The trait is governed by a gene, and this can be studied without necessarily knowing the biochemistry of the gene product. The geneticist, by appropriate mating experiments, can also work out a map of the various components of the nucleus (chromosomes) and can assign to a gene a definite place on that map. The spot on a chromosomal map occupied by a given gene is termed a *gene locus*. For some genes, there are only two possible alternatives. Take the example of a person's tendency to make offensive-smelling urine after eating asparagus. This is a genetic trait, and there are only two possibilities— you have it or you don't. These two alternatives at the gene level are termed *alleles*. In this particular case there are only two alleles at the gene locus concerned. However, there are other characteristics where there may be more alternatives. For example, a mouse may be white, black, brown, gray, and so forth. In this case there are multiple alleles, or a number of possible alternatives.

One complication arises when we recall that each cell in the body has components of both the mother and the father. The DNA of the human cell is compartmented into 46 separate bundles of DNA called chromosomes. There are 23 pairs, and of each pair, one is derived from the father and one from the mother. Every gene locus, with the exception of certain loci on the sex-determining chromosome pair, is represented twice. There is a good chance that the two chromosomes concerned will carry *different* alleles for a given gene; this is particularly the case for loci where there are multiple alleles. If a person carries a particular allele on both chromosomes, he is said to be *homozygous* for the gene concerned. If, as will happen more frequently, he carries a different allele on the two chromosomes, he is *heterozygous* at that gene locus. For certain gene loci, one allele can gain dominance over another, and be the only one expressed in the cell. This complication need not worry us in transplantation genetics, as the two alleles on the gene loci concerned are always codominant; that is, each expresses itself.

So far we have been speaking of characteristics governed by a single gene locus. In fact most characteristics of a human person are affected by a number of different genes. Qualities such as intelligence, height, weight, and beauty are not governed by a single gene; a number of quite different genes contribute. This is true also for the genes governing transplantation. It is not just one gene which governs the antigens appearing on the surface of a cell. In fact, one can show in the mouse that there are over 20 gene loci concerned in transplantation genetics, and the figure for man is probably similar. The technical word to describe these genes is *histocompatibility genes*. At many of these loci, there are not just two but eight or ten alleles. So you can see that the total number of different permutations and combinations of *histocompatibility genotypes* is quite astronomical, particularly when one bears in mind that most people will be heterozygous at most gene loci. In fact, no two people will be absolutely identical or perfectly matched with respect to histocompatibility. The only exceptions will be two identical twins. Just as a person's face or fingerprint is unique to him, so is his histocompatibility genotype.

All of this sounds terribly depressing from the standpoint of a surgeon who wants to perform organ transplants between two people. In fact, the picture is not quite so black. It has become clear that for all mammalian species, and probably for lower vertebrates as well, one particular cluster of genes is far more important than the others. This is known as the *major histocompatibility complex*, or MHC. The MHC is really a series of closely linked gene loci. No fewer than seven genes have been identified as belonging to it, and the likelihood is that there will be many more. However, because these genes sit relatively close together on the chromosome (ninth linkage group of chromosome 17 in the mouse), they tend to be inherited *en bloc*. The word *haplotype* is used to describe the particular allelic alternatives for the whole gene set which an individual inherits, and of course each person has two haplotypes, the paternal and the maternal (with occasional crossing over between the two). If mice or people are matched at the MHC loci, grafts will survive for long periods even though residual antigenic disparities persist at the other histocompatibility loci. Moreover, the residual immunological reaction against these weaker loci can be overcome readily with drugs or simple tolerance-inducing treatments. You can see already the practical importance of the MHC and the need for us to understand it, and there are even more fascinating complexities to come.

Experimental Transplantation in
Inbred Strains and Hybrids

You may well wonder how all this genetic knowledge about transplantation was gained. In all probability, the field would never have got off the ground were it not for the existence of inbred strains of animals, particularly mouse strains. To be useful, these have to be sufficiently inbred to resemble identical twins. At that stage, not only will every mouse accept a skin graft from every other mouse of the same sex within the strain, but every mouse will be *homozygous* at all histocompatibility loci. It is then possible to breed hybrids and these have taught us much about the ground rules governing transplantation. Consider for a moment simply the MHC loci of mice. Let us take two strains of mice, and let us for the sake of the present exercise pretend that the MHC were a simple gene instead of a linked cluster. Let us designate the haplotype of the first strain as A, and the second as B. As the strains are homozygous, both chromosomes will carry the same haplotype, and the genotype of the two strains can be written as AA and BB. Let us now mate an AA male with a BB female. Then *all* the progeny will be AB. The first filial generation, which we can term F_1, will *all* accept skin grafts from every other F_1 hybrid. They are just as histocompatible among each other as were the two parental strains. Now all histocompatibility genes are codominant, which means that both the A and the B antigen will be expressed on the surface of the AB cell. Consider now what happens when we try to graft skin from an F_1 hybrid back to one of the parents. Say we take AB skin and place it on the A parent. The A antigens will, of course, be recognized as "self" and do not cause immunization. But the B component is clearly foreign. It is a strong antigen, and the parent will throw its child's skin off quite promptly. What happens when we graft parental skin onto F_1 recipients? Whichever parent we use, the F_1 contains in its own body all the antigens of both parents. It recognizes either the A or the B skin as "self" and accepts the skin graft. If the parent and the F_1 are of different color, one can get quite impressive looking grafts, say, of white-haired skin on a brown mouse. This is illustrated in Figure 14–1.

Things get a little more interesting when we come to mate F_1s with F_1s, thereby creating the second filial or F_2 generation. Let us, for the moment, disregard all the histocompatibility genes except the MHC. Each F_1 will be AB, and we make an

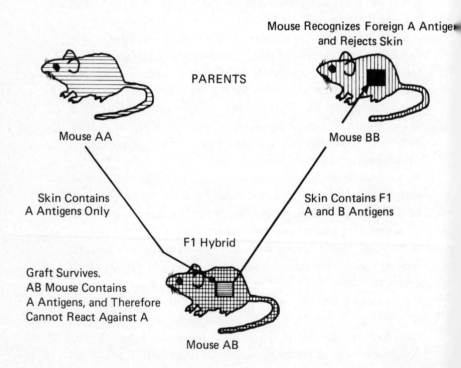

Figure 14–1. Skin graft behavior between parents and F_1 hybrids in inbred mice.

AB $\times$ AB F_2 hybrid. Clearly there will be three kinds of progeny: AA, AB, and BB. If one performs a large enough series of matings, the ratios of these will be 1:2:1. If we now try to graft skin from the original parent generation onto the hybrid, three out of four grafts on the average will take. If we choose AA skin, it will take on the AA and the AB mice, but not on the BB mice. Conversely, if you take F_2 skin and graft it onto either of the parents, only one in four will take. The AA would take an AA, but the AB and the BB would not.

Graft-versus-host Reactions

If one injects a graft of suspended cells containing lymphocytes into another animal, these are antigenic, and the graft is frequently rejected by a *host-versus-graft* reaction, the type of reaction we have been dealing with in the last two chapters. However, these lymphocytes, if alive, can also recognize antigens in the host and react against them. The result is termed a *graft-versus-host* reaction and really represents a form of civil warfare in the body. In most situations, the host will win out, as he has the full might of his whole system to fight against the cells that have been injected. However, there are conditions in which the host cannot defend himself. One is if he is very immature, with an immune system that is still in its infancy. Then the graft of lymphocytes can go on such a rampage that the host is killed. Another is if the immune system has been injured by some drug or treatment. From an experimental point of view, perhaps the most interesting is when, in inbred animals, parental lymphocytes are grafted onto an F_1 hybrid. The F_1 contains all the antigens of both parents. It is genetically tolerant of the parental graft and does not defend itself. The parent lymphocytes readily recognize one half of the antigens of the host F_1 animal (the half derived from its other parent) and mount a vigorous graft-versus-host reaction. This can frequently be lethal.

One interesting historical sidelight is that, but for a lucky chance, Sir Peter Medawar and his colleagues might never have discovered immunological tolerance (Chapter 12). They induced the tolerance by injections of living spleen cells into embryo mice. Fortunately, in the strain combination used, the graft-versus-host reaction was rather mild. Had a different pair of strains been tried, all the embryos would have been killed and the experiments might well have been abandoned.

Nomenclature of Grafting Procedures

With these genetic principles as a background, we are now in a position to introduce the technical terms describing various types of grafting procedures. A graft from some tissue of one's own body is called an *autograft*. If the donor and host are of identical genetic constitution, as in the case of inbred strains of mice or human identical twins, this is a *syngeneic homograft*. If the two members of the same species are genetically different this is an *allogeneic homograft*, or simply *allograft*. A graft performed from parent to F_1 or vice versa is referred to as a *semisyngeneic homograft*. Finally, a graft between two different species, such as rat to mouse or chimpanzee to man, is called a *xenograft*. The adjectives describing autografts and xenografts are *autochthonous* and *xenogeneic*: thus, "I performed an autochthonous split-thickness skin graft on that burnt child" or "The patient with the xenogenic kidney graft does not seem to be doing well." Familiarity with these terms will be helpful for readers who wish to delve deeper into the copious technical and semitechnical literature on transplantation. We will return to this topic and discuss it extensively in Chapter 17, but it might be appropriate to mention here that in mammals autochthonous and syngeneic grafts always take unless they are badly performed technically or some unforeseen accident occurs such as a blood clot or an infection. Allogeneic homografts face a host immune attack which can be overcome, under certain circumstances, by drugs, matching procedures, or both in combination. Xenografts take only under the most unusual circumstances.

The MHC in More Detail

The MHC is not just of importance in graft rejection. In fact, one of the most explosive facets of immunology today is tied up with the dawning realization that the MHC is important in lymphocyte interactions of both helper and suppressor nature; in the genetics of immune responsiveness; and for an understanding of how T lymphocyte receptors "see" antigens. In order to participate in this excitement, we have to look a litle harder at the MHC itself.

The key features for the mouse are schematized in Figure 14–2. Here, seven genes are seen as living close together. Two of these, the K and the D genes, which define the limits of the complex code for proteins which are present on the surface of every cell. These histocompatibility antigens are proteins of molecular weight 116,000, consisting of two disulfide-linked heavy chains of 46,000 and two noncovalently associated light chains of β_2-microglobulin, a molecule which shows amino-acid sequence homology with Ig. The K and D heavy chains are homologous to each other. Both are good, classical immunogens, and the sera of mice which have rejected allografts generally contain significant quantities of antibodies to them. For this reason, the K and D gene products are sometimes referred

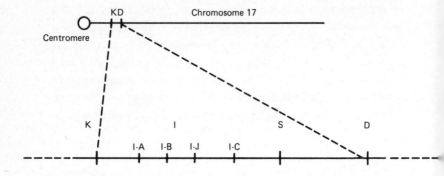

Figure 14–2. The major histocompatibility complex (MHC) in the mouse. This important chromosome region contains a cluster of linked genes that code for proteins important in cell interaction. The best understood are the histocompatibility antigens coded by K and D genes—it is these which cause foreign skin and kidney grafts to be rejected by the body. The I region is less well understood but the proteins coded by it are important for T cell–B cell cooperation and for other regulatory processes in the immune response.

to as SD or serologically determined antigens (a somewhat misleading name, as it is now evident that one can generate antibodies, though a little less readily, to other MHC gene products as well). The normal tissue-typing procedures carried out when attempts are made to match kidney graft donors and recipients rely heavily on antibodies of this sort.

The four sets of genes of the I region (to which more might well be added by the time this book is printed) are concerned with immune responsiveness and cell interactions. Within the IA and IC subregions of the gene complex there are genes coding for antigens which can lead to rejection of tissues, though these are not as powerful in eliciting the rejection reaction as K or D antigens. Also within these regions are antigens (perhaps the identical ones) which are particularly good at activating helper T cells and causing a good deal of lymphocyte division when lymphocytes of two different genotypes are co-cultured together. They have been referred to as LD or lymphocyte-determined antigens, in the present unfortunate and hopefully transient nomenclature. As we shall see in Chapter 15, the IA and IB subregions also code for genes (which may be structural or regulatory) that are important in determining how well an animal responds to certain antigens. The I region is involved in two other facets of the immune system. Genes within IA, IB, and IC code for glycoproteins known as Ia antigens that are present in high concentration on B lymphocytes; and I region gene products form part of both helper and suppressor factors manufactured by the appropriate T lymphocytes. It appears that the gene coding for suppressor factors lies in the newly defined IJ subregion, between IB and IC. Suppressor T cells carry this gene product on their surface, whereas helper T cells or B cells do not. But let me point out that the relationships between these very heterogeneous products, factors, and functions of the I region are still far from clear.

The S region is of less immediate concern to us. It codes for factors involved with the complement system. Its main importance has been in helping as a convenient marker in sorting out the above complexities.

T Cell Recognition and the "Altered Self" Concept

We saw in Chapter 4 that the question of T cell recognition of antigens is not quite straightforward. The clearest example of what I mean comes from an experiment reported recently by Drs. R. M. Zinkernagel and P. C. Doherty of Canberra, Australia. They were interested in the capacity of immunized

T lymphocytes to kill syngeneic cells which had been infected
with a virus, presumably through a direct union of the T cell
receptor for antigen with viral antigens present on the surface
of the infected cells. When these same antiviral killer T lymphocytes were placed in contact with allogeneic cells infected with
the same virus, surprisingly they failed to kill. This led to the
possibility that the T lymphocyte receptor saw not just viral
antigen but really the viral antigen in association with an MHC
self-antigen. In other words, the T cells might have a receptor
dictionary particularly fitted to recognizing variations of antigens associated with MHC products, or to see mainly "altered
self." When the restriction in antiviral killer capacity was investigated more closely, it turned out that genetic identity at either
K or D gene loci was sufficient to permit effective killing. Identity at any or all I region loci was not sufficient. This suggests
that killer T cells "see" antigens in association with K or D
antigens. In contrast, there is evidence that the T cells mediating
delayed hypersensitivity perceive antigenic determinants in close
association with the IA region gene product. Thus, different T
cell subsets may differ in which "altered self" component they
see.

The "altered self" model is not the only explanation for the
strange recognition capacities of T cells. It is possible that a
compound or linked recognition is required—an Ig-like receptor recognizing antigenic determinants and simultaneously
another, not yet identified T cell receptor recognizing the appropriate MHC product. This second reaction could be a "like-
like" interaction (e.g., K molecules linking up to adjacent,
identical K molecules) or a lock-and-key type recognition, in
which case one would have to postulate that T cells had "anti-
self" receptors on their surface. When this puzzle has been
sorted out, the function of the MHC and its products will be
much clearer.

We noted that the immunoglobulin genes evolved by gene
duplication, probably from an ancestral gene coding for a single

Ig domain of about 110 amino acids. The close homology between K and D gene products strongly suggests that these two genes also arose by duplication. At present, nothing is known of the amino-acid sequence of I gene products, but it is tempting to speculate that they will represent a series of homologous proteins as well. Perhaps the whole MHC represents a cluster of genes that arose from a single ancestral gene, the products of which perform various allied functions in cell interactions and recognition.

The MHC in man and other mammalian species contains a similar set of genes. There is one important difference, however, and that is that genes analogous with those of the I region lie not between K and D but to one side of them. The recognition of subcomponents of the I region in man has not yet moved as far as in the mouse, but at least two genes have been recognized—one coding for antigens present on every living cell and one for antigens present mainly on B lymphocytes. As far as tissue typing prior to transplantation is concerned, routine procedures concentrate on the equivalents of K and D antigens. But methods for typing at other loci are developing rapidly.

When scientists began inbreeding mice in the early part of the twentieth century, little did they realize that they were setting the stage for a major revolution in medical and surgical practice. It was not until the 1950s that the outlines of the genetic rules governing transplantation began to emerge, largely because of work in inbred mice. Not until the 1960s were these principles applied to man, and the spectacular success of human organ transplantation which began in that decade was certainly predicted by no one. The field of transplantation indicates very clearly the nexus between pure and applied research, and the mutual value of one to the other.

15

GENETICS OF ANTIBODY FORMATION

IT IS a central tenet of evolutionary theory that acquired characteristics cannot be inherited: the blacksmith does not pass on his bulging arm muscles to his sons. We have seen how immunological reactions of all kinds are very much acquired, reflecting each individual's history of exposure to antigens. This acquired memory cannot be passed on, except in the very limited sense of a mother's passing some antibodies to her infant via the placenta or in breast milk. What, then, do we mean by the genetics of antibody formation? Essentially, not the inheritance of actual immunity, but the inheritance of the capacity to mount an immune response. There are both quantitative and qualitative differences in the ways that individuals meet an antigenic challenge such as an infection, and, to a substantial degree, these differences are genetically determined. The nature of the response can have great medical significance, and the progressive unravelling of the genes controlling immunity is being watched closely by practicing physicians. The physiology of immune reactions is complex and so is their genetic control. These must be examined at various levels.

Nonspecific High and Low Responder Strains

When a randomly chosen, outbred group of mice (or people) is given an injection of a vaccine, and the antibody levels are measured a week or two later, there is a considerable variation in the amount which has been formed. All the individuals may be perfectly healthy, yet the highest responder may have ten times as much antibody as the lowest. Partly, this reflects the past immunological history of each adult and the amount of cross-reactive stimuli that have been previously encountered. However, if one now mates a low responder with a low responder, and a high responder with a high one, and continues the process through several generations, the two sets of progeny will each show a dispersion of values once again. But if the groups are sufficiently large, a statistical inheritance of high or low responsiveness will be seen. If this procedure is repeated over 20 generations, always mating the highest responders with the highest, the lowest with the lowest, quite marked differences emerge. There will be no overlap in the two dispersions: the best mouse in the low responder group will form less antibody than the worst in the high responder group.

This form of inherited quantitative difference in immune responsiveness is antigenically nonspecific. The mice respond well or poorly, whatever vaccine is given. Moreover, it is not traceable to a single gene or chromosomal area. Rather, it appears to be a multi-gene trait. In searching for mechanisms underlying the differences between high and low responder strains, two suggestions have emerged. The first is that the efficiency of the antigen-capturing structures and cells is variant, poor responses coinciding with inefficient antigen removal by macrophages. The second observation suggests that inherent cell division rates are slower in the low responders, a similar number of competent B cells being triggered but a slower division rate leading to much smaller clones. The experiments have been somewhat artificial. There does not appear to be much chance of such continuous selection for low immune responders occurring naturally.

Females *Are* the Stronger Sex

If a sufficiently large number of tests are done on normal adults, it is observed that females form more antibody than males. In a very large computer survey that Dr. G. L. Ada and I ran some years ago on our own pooled experiments in rats, the difference was nearly twofold on the average, not a very large difference given the wide variability in immune responsiveness, but statistically significant. It is possible that nature has programmed in this superiority to help females to cope with the special vulnerability associated with childbirth. Many autoimmune diseases are commoner in women than in men, and one cannot help wondering whether that is the price which had to be paid for a more reactive immune system.

Immunoglobulin Germ-Line, Gene-Associated Inheritance

We saw in Chapter 5 the fact that there was an array of genes coding for the variable portions of Ig light and heavy chains. Probably the set carried in the germ line is not huge, and somatic processes play an important part in generating the immunological repertoire. Nevertheless, the structure of the germ-line V genes provides the starting point for somatic diversification, and is thus very important in determining immune potential.

One clear way of demonstrating this fact is when mice are immunized against the haptenic molecule phosphoryl choline (PC). By a strange quirk, mice make far fewer antibody molecules containing λ light chains than κ light chains. In fact, λ makes up only 3 percent of the total Ig light-chain content of mouse serum. It is probable that there is only one germ line λ gene in the mouse. Of course, different inbred mice possess different allelic forms of this gene. Certain mouse strains possessing a particular λ allele in the germ line, the product of which is very good at recognizing PC, synthesize antibody that is almost all λ-containing on challenge with PC. Others, with a different allelic form of the λ gene, make mainly κ-containing antibodies, as is usual for mice.

Another example of the importance of germ-line V genes in steering the immune response is the inheritance of idiotypes. When an antigen of restricted heterogeneity, frequently a polymeric carbohydrate, is injected into an animal, the antibodies that appear may be predominantly of one or a very few clones. The combining sites of such homogeneous antibodies can be recognized by antisera made against them—so-called anti-idiotypic sera. When the progeny of such an animal are tested, they may make the identical idiotype as their parent, recognized by their reaction with the same anti-idiotype serum, or even through appropriate amino-acid sequence studies. A different animal, with a different genetic constitution, will make quite a different idiotype to the same antigen.

Obviously, this form of inheritance of immune responsiveness is specific for a particular antigen. It determines what kind of antibody, in terms of structure, an animal is likely to make when confronted with a given antigen. It is in that respect quite different to the other two forms of inheritance of immune responsiveness mentioned above.

MHC-linked Immune Response Genes

By far the most interesting aspect of the genetics of antibody formation is concerned with immune response genes linked to the major histocompatibility complex. This by now large and fashionable facet of immunology was first uncovered in the early 1960s through the use of synthetic protein antigens. We have mentioned several times that most protein antigens are mosaics of diverse antigenic determinants, and a total immune response against such a protein is a summation of the separate responses to the various determinants. This has a tendency to obscure genetic differences of a determinant-specific nature. An animal might be a high responder against determinant A, but a low responder to determinant B. If contrasted with another animal that is a low responder against determinant A but high against B, no net difference in antibody to the whole protein will be detected. However, if a protein is made synthetically out of only three or four amino acids, an antigen with a much lesser diversity of determinants results. One commonly used example is called TGAL, a copolymer consisting of a backbone of alanine and lysine residues, with side chains of glutamic acid and tyrosine. It was noted that when mice of various inbred strains were immunized against TGAL, they fell sharply into two groups. Some made a substantial amount of antibody, with the normal moderate variability in levels. Others made virtually no antibody at all. The quantitative differences can be a hundredfold. The responder or nonresponder status is a genetic trait: all mice of some genetic strains are responders, all mice of other genetic strains nonresponders. Moreover, a strain that is a responder against one particular synthetic polypeptide may be a nonresponder to another antigen. In other words, the immune response genes concerned are *antigen-specific*.

Two other startling facts were soon noted. First, the responsiveness or nonresponsiveness of a strain depended on its MHC genotype. If ten different mouse strains all shared the same MHC genotype, they would *all* be responders to some antigens, nonresponders to others. That is, the immune response genes were MHC-linked. We now know that they map within the I region of the MHC. Second, the nonresponsiveness of a strain could be readily overcome if the antigen concerned were hooked onto an immunogenic carrier. This proved that the B cells capable of making the relevant antibodies do exist within the nonresponder strains. What is lacking is a helper T cell capable of recognizing the synthetic antigen concerned. The defect in nonresponders is in the T cell compartment, and when the antigen is linked to a carrier against which helper T cells *can* be raised, then the B cells swing into action quite smartly.

A few years ago, this recognition of the T cell as the important target for the MHC-linked immune response genes appeared explicable in a simple way. The argument went as follows: T cells have a new, unknown kind of chemical recognition structure for antigens. A genetic nonresponder to antigen A is an animal in which the T cell receptor for A does not exist. The products of the I genes are simply the T cell receptors for antigens. Even before chemical knowledge about the T cell receptor accumulated, arguments could be raised against this view. The specificity of T cell recognition for antigen can be exquisitely good. For example, two chemically closely related haptens or two synthetic polypeptides differing in only one amino acid can readily be discriminated. This means T cells have an extensive recognition repertoire. If this is essentially different from the V gene system worked out for antibodies, then nature would have had to invent the immune system twice over—considered by most an unlikely possibility. Recent evidence showing identical idiotypes on T and B cell receptors, and other chemical evidence, make it virtually certain that the T cell receptor site for antigens is a V gene product. This leaves us in somewhat of a mess in understanding the MHC-linked immune response genes. The most likely bet is that they code for molecules important in cell-cell interaction, e.g. for B cell receptors for T cell helper or suppressor factors. The real puzzle is how these can be antigen-specific. There have recently been claims that the specificity of immune response genes is not as great as that of antibodies, and it could be that the diversity of immune response gene products is much less than that of V regions.

A further complication has recently arisen. It turns out that responsiveness to some antigens is controlled by more than one gene in the I region. Genetic tests known as gene complementation studies have shown that the progeny of two nonresponders can sometimes be responders, and further analysis puts this down to the presence of two genes, one in the IA subregion and the other probably in IB. The possession of a responder allele at either gene can make the animal a responder. Moreover, again within the I region, specific suppressor genes, distinct from the regular immune response genes, have been identified. It will be some time till we have a satisfactory understanding of these.

Immune Response Genes and Human Disease

I might have been tempted to omit reference to this rapidly moving but still somewhat turbid area of immune response genes, were it not for one observation. This is that the genes may be of extreme importance in some human diseases. It now turns out that certain diseases of obscure causation are far more common in people of a particular MHC genotype than in other people. The most extreme example of this is a debilitating chronic arthritic condition of the spine known as ankylosing spondylitis. With rare exceptions, this occurs *only* in people bearing the MHC antigen known as HLA B27. Noteworthy associations of important diseases such as multiple sclerosis, celiac disease, psoriasis, and many others with particular MHC alleles have been reported. One hypothesis that commands much support is the following. These diseases could be caused by a virus or other infectious agent such as the peculiar bacterial forms known as mycoplasmas. The agent for multiple sclerosis might even be a commonly occurring one like measles virus. Most people cope successfully with an infection, but a few, possessing a nonresponder genotype towards it, fail to mount an adequate T cell attack. The virus therefore persists— not in the bloodstream, but within cells, causing a chronic disease. Another view holds that these diseases are autoimmune in nature, and that the possession of certain immune response genes guides the system towards this abnormal responsiveness. So far, most of the testing in humans has been for the genotype of the equivalents of K and D, and such few tests as are available for the more directly relevant region (the analogue of I) suggest associations will be even closer.

This chapter and the tail end of the last may well strike you as the most difficult portions of this book. The reason is this: it is not easy to popularize when certain essential features of nature's design are still unclear. At the moment, the MHC contains the key to a thousand linked puzzles that are at the very forefront of academic immunology. The sessions dealing with it and related topics at international meetings cause heated and prolonged debate. There are aspects where the penny has not quite dropped. When it does (as certainly will be the case before our third edition!), the probability is that nature's plan will be revealed as very elegant yet quite simple. The apparent cumbersomeness of the present picture is due to our limitations, not those of evolution! My hope is that your struggle through an area that has not yet been completely assimilated into the established corpus of knowledge may have given you some inkling of how science works, and how researchers themselves must struggle and even flounder to arrive at the truth.

16

IMMUNITY AND
CLINICAL MEDICINE

In the fields of biology and medicine, a great deal of nonsense is talked about pure versus applied research. This can, in fact, do quite serious harm. There are certainly some people in universities who regard any experiment which has a motive beyond "knowledge for knowledge's sake" as somehow inferior. Conversely, in business and political circles, there are certain anti-intellectual elements that spoof any endeavor which does not lead to guaranteed practical results in a predictable time. These divisive voices are in the minority, but they help to perpetuate misconceptions and create tensions to the detriment of science and the progress of mankind. Those who have immersed themselves deeply into modern science know that there is a continuum between the most basic probing into the abstruse realms of theory and an endeavor as clearly applied as a planned evaluation of a new drug. All intermediate stages exist; all are equally important and useful; all will progress together.

The great pity is that even people who should know better allow themselves to become embroiled in semantic arguments and polarized positions. For example, when the famous Rothschild report came out in the United Kingdom, its actual recommendations were for a small percentage of research funds to go directly to departments of state for the pursuit of applied research endeavors related to priority areas chosen by the government. It is difficult to quarrel violently with such a plan, yet the report caused a furor, both because it used injudicious phrases such as "scientific roulette" (describing fundamental, investigator-initiated research) and because many immediately saw it as the thin edge of the wedge threatening scientific freedom. In the event, it is apparent some years after the adoption of the report in the United Kingdom that no very dreadful changes have resulted in research.

Another very clear point is that cross-reactions between the more basic and the more applied fields are constantly occurring and are increasingly important. One of the greatest benefits of the space race, an example of applied science, has been the development of a large variety of materials, instruments, and findings of great use in universities and in many distant fields of research. Out of the revolution in molecular biology, which is the highlight of basic biological science in this half-century, may one day flow treatments for congenital defects and even cancer. In neither example is the fundamental value of the work, applied and basic, respectively, judged by the extent of the spinoff into the opposite arena. In both cases, the nexus develops spontaneously and efficiently in a free society.

From its very beginnings, immunology has been an outstanding example of the interwoven nature of so-called pure and applied science. Louis Pasteur made no secret of his desire to achieve important practical goals, but his work on the nature of putrefaction and infection, which destroyed the "spontaneous generation" theory of microbial life, must rank as basic scientific work of the highest order. The other early giants of the field—Bordet, Gengou, von Behring, Koch, Ehrlich, and Metchnikoff—represent a spectrum of interests and disciplines, and each would have rejected categorization into either theoretical or practical classes. Landsteiner was the purest of scientists, yet his work led directly to the introduction of successful blood transfusion, one of the earliest and great triumphs of scientific medicine. This general trend has continued to the present day. Certainly, immunology numbers among its exponents chemists and physical chemists who would feel very lost in a hospital ward; and physicians and surgeons who would pale with fright if asked to operate a high-speed ultracentrifuge or to make sense out of an amino-acid sequence. However, it includes a great majority of people who know a little about most aspects of the spectrum and a lot about a particular facet. Most important of all, the discipline runs the whole distance, and in its path frequently acts as a force that illuminates, fertilizes, and unifies.

So far, we have dealt mainly with antibody formation and cellular immunity in normal animals and human beings. In the succeeding chapters we will be turning to an examination of the role of immunology in disease states. This is a vast subject, and only the most outstanding examples will be considered. Broadly speaking, we can look at the subject under three headings. First, there are disease states which are fundamentally due to unwanted, unhealthy, immune responses. Second, there are cases in which there is nothing obviously wrong with the immune system, but we want to manipulate it in some way to prevent or cure a nonimmunological condition. Third, there are occasions which involve immunological science, not in the treatment but in the diagnosis of a disease. In the first group, we include allergies, hypersensitivity, and autoimmune diseases. These are dealt with in Chapters 18 and 19. The second group embraces all attempts at specific immunization to prevent infectious diseases, and conditions in which we wish to lower the immune response, as in organ transplantation, or strengthen it, as in certain approaches to the cancer problem. Various aspects relating to this group will be dealt with in Chapters 17, 20, and 21. It remains here to dispose briefly of the other aspects of this second group, and of the third problem.

Infectious Diseases Not Yet Preventable by Vaccination

There are two types of infectious disease in which immunization has been spectacularly successful. The first is the prevention of virus diseases which spread widely through the body. These include smallpox, yellow fever, poliomyelitis, measles, and mumps. Vaccination against these is safe and practically 100 percent effective. The second is in the prevention and treatment of bacterial diseases where the invading microbe makes a strong poisonous substance which travels in the blood and exerts a destructive effect at some site in the body distant from where the infection actually is. Good examples are tetanus (or lockjaw) and diphtheria. In tetanus, the bacteria multiply in a wound, but send their poisons to cause spasms in muscles which may be quite distant. In diphtheria, the microbes grow to form a thick membrane which coats the tonsils and surrounding throat area, but the toxin travels to the heart and makes its action weak and flabby. Both these conditions can be prevented by regular injections of an altered poison which retains the necessary antigenic groupings but is no longer toxic. These substances, called toxoids, are usually injected several times in early life, and at intervals thereafter to maintain the immune state. These toxoids do not give an absolute degree of safety. An occasional case of tetanus or diphtheria has been recorded in an immunized person, but these are quite rare and usually very mild. If a case of one of these diseases is diagnosed, and usually this will be in an unimmunized individual, antibody from another human, or if that is not available, from a horse, can be injected. The effect will depend on the degree of damage which had already occurred before the treatment was given. Usually, if a toxin has already poisoned the action of a given nerve or muscle cell, this cell's function will not be affected by giving passive antibody. All one can hope to do is prevent the poison from reaching cells that are not yet damaged. So, everything depends on early diagnosis and treatment. Passive immunization can be bitterly disappointing if given too late, as the still high mortality in cases of tetanus shows.

Some immunization procedures employing whole, killed bacteria as immunogens are widely used. These include vaccinations for whooping cough, typhoid, paratyphoid, cholera, and plague. Broadly speaking, these vaccines are not as uniformly satisfactory as the above two categories. Disease incidence is significantly lowered, but not abolished, if exposure occurs. One has the feeling that more research into the most important antigens is needed, and then greater effort will have to be expended to extract the antigens in a purer form. Many people will be familiar with the sore arms that typhoid shots give. The arms would be much less sore and the vaccines more effective if purified antigens were used, provided it had been proven that antibodies against the particular antigen used could prevent infection. In part, it may not be the vaccine which is at fault, but the natural habitat of the organism. If a microbe lives in the gut or the lining of the throat and windpipe, it is not exposed to as high and consistent a concentration of antibodies as if it had to negotiate a long journey through the bloodstream. This consideration applies even more to virus diseases such as influenza, in which the virus lives largely in superficial mucous membrane cells. Flu vaccines can cause quite good antibody levels to appear in the blood, but often the amount present on the surface of the throat is not enough to prevent infection. Another problem with flu is that there are so many antigenic variants; immunity against one strain affords no protection against another.

One is often asked: "What about a vaccine for the common cold?" Again, the answer is that there are so many different viruses capable of causing coughs and runny noses that vaccination against all the varieties present in a community at a particular time is just not practicable. If it were, the immunity given would be quite short-lived, and shots would have to be frequently repeated. There is no doubt that immunity against these types of viruses is not a total pipe dream. For example, when a group of men go down to spend a year in Antarctica, where one would think that colds and flu might abound, it is a very common experience to find that for the entire period there, the men are quite healthy. They quickly become immune to whatever viruses others in the group are carrying, and all harmful organisms die out for want of a nonimmune host. When they return home, however, even the penetrating sunshine will not prevent a wave of minor coughs and colds because there will not be immunity to all the variants present in a large community.

A further problem which besets preventive medicine is a group of diseases in which we know a virus is at work, but it has either never been grown or else is not yet available in sufficiently pure form to make a completely satisfactory vaccine. Infectious hepatitis is in the former category; rabies or hydrophobia in the latter, though very recent work may have solved this problem. A very formidable problem exists also for bacteria that are hard to grow, such as leprosy. The absence of any form of vaccine for gonorrhea or syphilis presents further challenges for bacterial experts. One sometimes feels that these highly practical problems are not getting the quality of attention that they deserve. It is true that most of the conditions are curable by modern drugs, but an immunological approach could have important advantages. For example, it might be possible to create such a high proportion of resistance in the population that the microbe runs out of hosts and dies out. This is known as "herd immunity," which begins to be a significant factor when about three-quarters of a community are immune. Furthermore, as antibiotic-resistant strains become more common, public health thinking may swing back more to immunization programs.

The immunological approach to parasitic diseases, though still remote, is of such immense public health importance that we shall examine it separately in Chapter 21.

Immunological Methods in Diagnosis

One aspect of immunology with direct clinical implications is the use of immunological methods in diagnosis. Frequently it is important to eliminate a past or present infection as a cause of trouble in a difficult case. Here antibodies to particular bacteria present in the serum may give the clue to the diagnosis. Delayed hypersensitivity tests reveal portions of a person's past infectious history, as with the tuberculin tests. A completely different aspect of this problem is where sensitive techniques used for immunity work have been brought over directly to measure concentrations of substances present in very small amounts in the serum. For instance, many hormones present in very low amounts can be detected readily by means of their capacity to combine with antiserum, using a variety of tricks involving radioactive tracers. This may allow diagnosis of a hormone deficiency. Finally, antibody tests are very important in describing a person's genetic constitution. Witness the use of antibodies to detect specific blood groups and transplantation antigens.

Apart from diagnosis of the ailments of individuals, antibody tests are very important in epidemiology. If a scientist or public health official needs to know the prevalence of a particular disease in a community, one of the best ways is to search for the presence of antibodies or cellular immunity. Such sero-epidemiological studies are of special importance in countries where planners need to know the diseases of highest public health priority.

Diverse other facets of immunology impinge on the clinic, and each passing year sees more implications for practical medicine emerging. All of these are important, but none has caught the imagination of the public as much as the subject matter in the next chapter. Organ transplantation, particularly kidney transplantation, has a Brave-New-World flavor which has gained it almost too much prominence. We must now turn to this subject and to the other vital medical advances in immunology.

17

ORGAN
TRANSPLANTATION

Whale individuals may dream of personal immortality, nature's design on this earth has, from the beginning, depended on an inevitable cycle of birth, growth, reproduction, senescence, and death. Perhaps this is not a sine qua non of biological systems. Who can tell whether there may not be forms of life in other parts of the universe where evolution has not rested on survival of the fittest, where a permissive environment has allowed the development of life forms that grow without dividing, or persist without change? Certainly this is not possible on this earth. Our view of biology in the twentieth century is dominated by the theories of Charles Darwin. We accept almost intuitively that time and constant change are parameters of life; and after appropriate education, that essentially random copying errors in the replication of DNA molecules are the root source of variation and progress in the development of species. The copying errors can occur and give rise to expression only if cells and animals multiply. Moreover, the occasional superior being can gain dominance only in a setting of competition. If there were no struggle for survival, the odd advantageous mutation would be drowned out by a horde of neutral and deleterious mutations; evolution in the sense that we know it would be impossible. Thus, presumably at some very early stage in the evolution of species on this planet, death entered the world as the one inevitable consequence of life.

If death cannot be prevented, what is the central purpose of medical science? Not to make people live forever, but to ensure that the maximum possible percentage of human beings born into the world reach the biblical life span with a minimum of intervening disease. In old age, the purpose shifts subtly to a reasonable prolongation of life, relief of suffering, assistance to failing faculties, and maintenance of human dignity. It is not the role of medical science to confer a biologically impossible immortality. If we keep these concepts in perspective, we are ready for an adult and responsible look at the role of organ transplantation in human health.

Many deaths in people over 70 years are due to diseases that are widely diffused through the body. Hardening of the arteries (arteriosclerosis) and spreading cancer are the two most common, but there are many other examples. In younger people, multiple-organ diseases are also common, but there is still a large group of serious disorders in which essentially only one organ has gone wrong. The commonest cause of death in middle-aged men, for example, is a heart attack. This is due to the occlusion of a blood vessel bringing oxygen to the heart muscle. Sometimes, the disease which leads to blockage in the blood vessel is widespread through the body, but often it is practically confined to the small arteries supplying the heart. The whole person dies because of malfunction of one working part. There are other serious, common disorders which do not kill quickly but impair health and shorten life. Among these is diabetes, which is due to poor function of certain cells in the pancreas. A number of intermediate situations exist, in which a disease at first causes few symptoms, but as more and more of the particular organ concerned becomes involved, trouble appears and death can follow quite swiftly. Cirrhosis of the liver and various forms of chronic nephritis (kidney disease) are good examples. It is to disorders such as the above groups that organ transplantation is most relevant. The concept involves substitution of a good organ, usually from a recently deceased person, for the diseased, worn-out one. If it were possible to use all the healthy organs of all people who died from whatever cause to replace effectively the diseased organs of sick people, the savings in human life and suffering would be quite incalculable. We are a very long way from that goal, but still closer to it than anyone would have dreamed possible as recently as 1960.

Immunosuppression in Human Organ Transplantation

We learned in Chapter 14 that, apart from identical twins, no two people are alike in their histocompatibility genes. Therefore, any organ transplant from one person to another has to face the cellular immunity attack of the host. This will vary in intensity depending on the detailed differences between the donor and the host in their antigenic constitution. However, it will always be present. This is the major factor limiting the advance of organ transplantation as the answer to innumerable human ills. There are two broad ways by which we can confine the intensity of immune rejection of grafts to tolerable limits. The first is an artificial suppression of the immune response by drugs; the second, an attempt to minimize histoincompatibility of donor and host by genetic matching procedures. A third way would be still more desirable: to induce a state of immunological tolerance specific for the antigens of the particular graft, and especially towards MHC antigens. While much research today aims at achieving this, no method has reached the stage of clinical acceptability.

Treatment directed towards reducing the immune attack to an antigen is referred to as immunosuppression. There are three types of treatment that we must consider. The first is a group of hormone-like drugs called corticosteroids that resemble in their action the cortisone produced by cells in the cortex of the adrenal gland. Prednisone and prednisolone are probably the most widely used members of this group of drugs. The steroids damp down immune mechanisms in a variety of ways. They have a profound *anti-inflammatory* power, that is, they damp down the inflammation which normally follows any immunological encounter within the body. In high concentration, they can actually lead to destruction of some lymphocytes, markedly depleting the thymic cortex and lowering blood lymphocyte levels. They are membrane-active drugs and may interfere in some aspects of immune triggering. In acute immunological episodes, such as severe allergic reaction to a bee sting, or very severe asthma, corticosteroids can be literally lifesaving. In organ transplantation, they remain a powerful sheet anchor. Unfortunately, all of these strong effects require doses of drugs that raise blood concentrations to a far higher level than is normal. This is not too serious when a single dose is given, but can lead to profound side effects if the high doses are maintained for a long time. One effect is very common. The person who takes cortisone for several weeks or longer develops a characteristic puffiness of the cheeks and the side of the face. This moon-faced look is quite characteristic, and most doctors would spot a cortisone-taker as soon as the person walked through the door. It is particularly distressing for young girls or women patients. Other side effects, also reasonably common, include softening of the bones and development of peptic ulcers. For these reasons, it is every doctor's wish to keep cortisone doses as low as possible, and, if high doses are necessary to get a patient over an emergency, then to use these over as short a period as possible.

While cortisone alone was used in human organ transplants, the success rate was relatively low. It improved greatly when a drug called azathioprine was developed; this was first used in human beings in 1962. It is typical of a group of drugs which were first developed for the treatment of cancer. The central purpose of these drugs is to interfere with processes essential for cell division. Naturally, if all cell division in the body were to cease, death would result. Many of the body's systems depend on constant cell renewal. The skin, the hair follicles, the mucous membranes, and all the cells of the blood depend on constant replenishment of cells through the process of division.

How, then, can a drug like azathioprine be helpful? This depends on two facts. First, not all cells divide at the same rate, and those systems depending on rapidly dividing cells will be more severely affected by treatment with these drugs than tissues in which cell division is slower. This is the rationale of the use of such cell-division poisons in cancer treatment as, on the average, cancer cells divide more rapidly than normal cells. Of the body's different functions, none depends more intimately on rapid cell division than the immune response. Therefore, immune responses can be greatly reduced by doses of cell-division poisons considerably smaller than those which would impair the integrity of the skin or the intestinal lining. The second consideration is that not all dividing cells are influenced to exactly the same degree by a particular drug. Some drugs hit the hair follicles more than others; some have a special tendency to depress bone marrow function. Azathioprine has been chosen for immunosuppression because it tends to hit cells of the lymphoid system harder than it does any other type of dividing cell. In carefully chosen doses, it can depress immune responses while allowing adequate amounts of red cells and granulocytes to be made. Fortunately, it can block cellular immunity without disturbing hair growth or intestinal function.

While azathioprine has turned out to be a remarkably safe drug when intelligently used, it is neverthelesss vital to monitor patients regularly for harmful side effects.

The best results in clinical immunosuppression are achieved when cortisone-like drugs and azathioprine are used in combination rather than separately. As the mode of action is different, the toxic effects are not additive, but the immunosuppressive effects are. The combined approach is standard throughout the world in kidney graft centers. Physicians are particularly pleased that azathioprine can allow them to get away with much lower doses of corticosteroids; it has a steroid-sparing effect. The dosage of each drug must be carefully adjusted by the physician in charge for each particular case. It usually starts off quite high in the immediate postoperative period, and is then gradually reduced. At intervals, the lymphocytes seem to muster themselves from defeat and mount a sudden counterattack. This troop movement can be spotted by the alert physician. It is termed a "rejection crisis." The treatment is immediate administration of much larger doses of the immunosuppressive drugs. These are given for a few days in doses that would be quite toxic if maintained for long, but which are relatively safe over short periods under strict medical supervision in hospital. This often allows the rejection crisis to be rapidly overcome. Rejection crises are most common in the first six months after a transplant, and relatively rare after a year.

In 1965, a third agent was introduced for clinical use in transplantation which can serve as an adjunct to the above two groups of drugs. This is anti-lymphocyte serum, or ALS. The principle on which ALS therapy is based is the following: If immune responses are based on lymphocytes, does it not make much better sense to inhibit the lymphocytes directly than to diminish cell division in general? ALS is made by taking human lymphocytes and injecting them into a horse or other suitable animal. The horse will make antihuman lymphocyte antibodies.

Unfortunately, it makes antibodies against other human antigens present in trace amounts in the lymphocyte suspensions. These are largely removed by a process called absorption, before ALS is used. However, it is not usually possible to eliminate them completely, and so ALS can have some toxic side effects. Its main action is on T lymphocytes, which, as an overall population, recirculate more extensively than B lymphocytes and are thus harder hit by an agent introduced into the circulation. ALS is now usually marketed as ALG, the globulin fraction which contains all the antibodies. Its main usefulness in most centers has been in the management of rejection crises, where it can be most helpful. Few centers have used ALG routinely for long-term immunosuppression, although some that do have reported a lowering in the number of rejection crises, and of drug dosage. Apart from contaminating antibodies (such as anti-red cell antibodies or anti-platelet antibodies) in ALG, the worst problem is the development by the patient of antibodies to ALG itself. After all, horse or rabbit globulin is a foreign antigen in man. When antibodies are developed, the risks in man include severe inflammatory reactions at the site of injection, fever, deposition of immune complexes in the kidneys, not to speak of the obvious fact that the anti-ALG antibodies will lead to its elimination and thus lower its effect on lymphocytes. These nasty side effects can be lessened or even eliminated by first inducing immunological tolerance to the foreign globulin in the patient. This can be done by giving a large and carefully de-aggregated intravenous dose of *normal* (non-ALG) globulin from the species concerned to the patient some days before commencing ALG.

Immunological Tolerance and Human Transplantation

It will be apparent that all of the above treatments share one grave disadvantage. Not only is the patient's immune attack against the graft diminished, but also his capacity to mount any other sort of immune attack is impaired to an equal degree. Therefore, graft patients are very susceptible to infections, particularly in the postoperative months when dosage of immunosuppressants is highest. This is the biggest single cause of death in kidney graft recipients. It would be very advantageous if there were methods of turning off the immune response against the antigens of the graft, while leaving immune responses to all other antigens, including microorganisms, in good shape. This would be accomplished if a stable state of immunological tolerance (Chapter 12) were induced in the host toward the histocompatibility antigens of the graft. This can be accomplished in experimental animals, but not yet in man. As our knowledge of purified transplantation antigens increases, it might be possible to prepare fractions or antigen fragments which cause tolerance instead of an immune response. This is one of the great aims of current transplantation research. In fact, while the lymphocyte attackers are kept at bay by immunosuppression, some form of accommodation between graft and host does occur. This is obvious by the diminishing incidence of rejection crises and the lower doses of drugs which can be used. However, this is not strictly immunological tolerance. For example, if a kidney graft has been in place for a year, and the patient or animal is now on relatively low doses of immunosuppression, a skin graft from the same donor can still be rejected briskly. The exact mechanism is still rather obscure, but the practical outcome of "learning to live together" is hopeful, making long-term survival of the graft possible without excessive therapy.

Matching in Human Transplantation

The complexity of the histocompatibility loci, discussed in Chapter 14, renders perfect matching of donor and host impossible. However, superb results *can* be achieved in the case of siblings carrying identical MHC haplotypes. Consider two parents who, not being inbred, are likely to be heterozygous at the various MHC loci. Let us ignore the small but real possibility of a genetic crossing-over within the MHC, and suppose the haplotype is inherited en bloc. If the father is AB, and the mother CD, four types of children can result, namely AC, AD, BC, and BD. If a particular sick person with a destroyed kidney types BD, using appropriate leucocyte typing reagents, the transplant surgeon will look to see if there is a sibling also typing BD, who (if possessed of two normal kidneys and otherwise healthy) could act as a volunteer kidney donor. It is also essential to match for compatibility of the major ABO blood groups. If the match is good in those two respects, identity at the minor histocompatibility loci is much less important. In fact, such MHC-identical grafts have been enormously satisfying, requiring minimal immunosuppression and in general having no rejection crises.

Life is not so simple in the case of unrelated cadaver transplants, because the MHC is a compound gene locus and at least four genes contribute to antigenicity. If donor and host are (as they generally will be) heterozygous at all four, there are eight factors requiring to be matched up. Moreover, typing is only a simple, straightforward matter with respect to the SD loci (see Chapter 14) and methodologies for typing at the LD loci are only now coming forward. There is some controversy about whether it is in fact worthwhile to attempt to match donor and host for the two main SD loci. In practice, it is rare to be able to achieve a "full house" match (four antigens identical between

donor and host) even for these, and usually one has to settle
for three or even less. While some groups stoutly maintain that,
statistically, transplants do better with fewer mismatched antigens, the largest published series fails to substantiate this view.
The position will have to be reviewed when LD typing becomes
more commonplace.

Kidney Transplantation

By far the most progress has been made in the transplantation
of a single organ—the kidney. At the time of the First International Congress of the Transplantation Society, held in Paris
in mid-1967, 1,400 cases of renal transplantation in man had
been reported to the kidney transplant registry maintained in
Boston. In the nine years following that, a further 25,000 transplants have been performed and half of these otherwise doomed
patients are still alive. A number of factors conspired to make
the kidney a logical target for the early exploration of the
potential of organ transplantation in man. The development of
an artificial kidney played an important role. This is an instru-
ment which rids the blood of unwanted waste material in much
the same way that a real kidney does. It requires that the blood
of the patient should circulate through the machine for periods
of eight to twelve hours. This means that blood containing all
the waste matter that has built up over a period of kidney failure
is taken from an artery in the patient's arm by means of a tube
which stays in place through the whole cleansing procedure. A
special anti-clotting agent is used to prevent blockage. By means
of an auxiliary pump, the blood is passed over a series of
membranes where it is purified. It returns to a vein in the
patient's arm, and thence back to the heart. This artificial
kidney procedure is termed hemodialysis, and was first devised
to cope with patients whose own kidneys had undergone some

acute shock and had failed temporarily but were suffering from reversible damage. There also exist many conditions where both kidneys become irrevocably destroyed by progressive disease. These form the group in whom transplants are necessary. The artificial kidney plays a vital role in helping them to get fit for operation. People with advanced kidney disease are frequently wasted, anemic, and in very poor general shape. Repeated hemodialysis and good hospital care bring them up to the standard of health necessary before major surgery. Frequently, a patient can be maintained on an artificial kidney for many months prior to transplantation. This requires two hemodialysis procedures per week.

A second reason for choosing the kidney for transplant work is that excellent techniques for performing the delicate surgery have been worked out. As specialized operations go, grafting a kidney is a relatively simple procedure. Pioneers in this area in the early 1950s were Drs. Joseph Murray, John Merrill, and David Hume at the Peter Bent Brigham Hospital in Boston. Since their early work, some technical improvements have been made, and hundreds of surgeons in all the developed countries are expert in the procedure. The operation is outlined in Figure 17–1. It requires two surgical teams, one operating on the donor and one on the recipient. Even if the donor is a cadaver rather than a living volunteer, full surgical asepsis must be used. The donor kidney is removed with its artery and vein carefully dissected free and intact. Also, the tube draining urine from the kidney to the bladder (the ureter) must be preserved. Then, the kidney is placed into the abdomen of the recipient, usually in the lower right corner. The artery is connected with one of the main branches of the aorta; the vein is joined to a large vein at the back of the abdomen; and the end of the ureter is implanted into the bladder. Care is taken to minimize the period during which the donor kidney has no blood pumping through it. Any period of absent oxygenation longer than an hour or two damages the donor kidney. Frequently, the

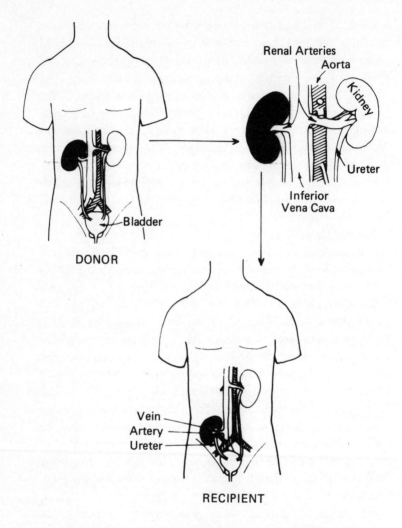

Figure 17–1. The operation of kidney transplantation.

patient's own, destroyed kidneys are removed; they serve no useful function and often help to cause a high blood pressure state. The patient is best rid of them.

There are several other reasons that we can list for the pre-eminence of kidney grafts as the pacesetters in the transplant revolution: chronic kidney disease is all too common and often fatal; it makes good sense to consolidate knowledge around one procedure rather than to fragment the surgical research efforts into too many avenues; the kidney is a paired organ, and a person can function adequately with only one, a consideration which makes it possible to use human volunteers on occasion; and kidney sufferers are often young and their other organs quite healthy. We must also not forget the importance of example and apprenticeship in medical education. The superb lead that has been given by several pioneer groups in kidney transplantation has been an example which has captured the imagination of the whole world, and a skilled army of doctors has been trained by the pioneers and their students.

Results of Kidney Transplantation, 1977

As with any surgical procedure, much depends on the expertise and experience of the team in charge. The following generalizations apply to major groups, usually at well-equipped teaching hospitals. Transplants in identical twins have a 97 percent chance of success, with only a very occasional technical disaster. Transplants between MHC-identical siblings rate a better than 90 percent chance of good long-term functioning. Further to that, the best groups report 75–80 percent success in cases where matching procedures and living volunteers are used, and 60–70 percent where cadavers donate the kidneys. In all cases, the maximum danger period is in the first six months after transplantation. If the graft survives this period its chances for long-term functioning are good. Of course, a certain small drop-off occurs in later years as well, and one definite risk is that the transplant may, over the years, develop the same disease as destroyed the original kidneys. Still, a significant proportion of patients will enjoy the same fate as John Riteris, who was presented to the Sixth International Congress of the Transplantation Society in New York in 1976 as the longest survivor of kidney transplantation—hale and hearty 17 years after his operation. Moreover, even the disaster of an acute graft rejection is now often overcome. The rejected kidney is surgically removed, the patient is put back on the artificial kidney, and awaits his or her turn for a further transplant. Unquestionably, kidney transplants are here to stay—not yet a perfect triumph but still one of the major achievements of modern scientific medicine.

Heart Transplantation

When Dr. Christiaan Barnard performed the first human heart transplant in 1967, using a technique developed by Drs. Norman Shumway and Richard Lowther at Stanford University, California, he created a world furor. Since then, 316 heart transplants have been performed (to September, 1976), but only 63 patients are alive. This 20 percent success rate is certainly much lower than that of kidney grafts. Among the reasons are the following. First, obviously only cadavers and not living relatives can be used as donors. Second, as this is a desperate procedure, the recipients are in very poor condition at the time of operation. Third, the blood vessels of the heart appear to be very susceptible to immunological attack by the host. Fourth, there is nothing comparable to the artificial kidney to help the patient through a rejection crisis. Finally, there is no doubt that the more widespread use of the procedure, and thus the building up of greater clinical experience, has been limited through very legitimate ethical concerns. It has become clear that our definitions of death are by no means all that certain. For example, people whose respiration and heartbeat have stopped can be resuscitated, and even a cessation of electrical activity in the brain has, very occasionally, been followed by prolonged survival (though never a return to normal life). It is best to be very conservative in defining death, and therefore it is likely that heart transplantation will remain an unusual operation.

Liver Transplantation

Chronic liver disease is not uncommon. While about half the cases of chronic scarring of the liver, or cirrhosis, are due to alcoholism, the other half are the end result of a variety of liver diseases, including virus infections or autoimmune diseases. For the destroyed liver, there is no treatment comparable to hemodialysis, even though exchange blood transfusions can be helpful in tiding patients over an *acute* liver episode.

There is one major difference between liver transplants and the operations so far considered. The operation itself is fiendishly difficult and demanding. Probably no more than half a dozen teams in the world have built up sufficient experience to tackle it with confidence. As in the case of heart transplants, these groups have been heartened by some spectacular successes, but the overall figures lag behind those of kidney grafts.

Transplantation of Other Organs

One field of transplantation that has been a little disappointing is the one that started the whole area of development—skin transplantation. Many people die of severe burns, and a good proportion of these are children. The main causes of death are shock, fluid loss, and the lack of a protective coating over so much of the body's surface. Burn victims who survive are usually cruelly scarred. By far, the best treatment would be skin from a cadaver. However, skin graft rejection is such a vigorous process that it is extremely difficult to turn off. Moreover, azathioprine and cortisone would be very dangerous drugs in a patient acutely ill from severe burns. It seems that the extensive lymphatic drainage which develops brings foreign antigens to the lymph nodes in such force that eventual rejection is inevitable. Even so, skin allografts can be a useful first-aid dressing in cases of severe burns. Later, autografts of thin, split layers of skin can be applied from a healthy area of the patient's own body. The depth of these grafts is so adjusted by the plastic surgeon that the donor site has enough cells left to recover without scarring, and the graft itself contains enough cells from the deeper skin layers to take and continue to grow.

There was an unfortunate episode in transplantation research when Dr. William Summerlin reported that culturing skin in tissue culture for three weeks removed its capacity to be rejected. This experiment turned out to be irreproducible, and fraudulent behavior was detected. It is true that submitting tissues to culture will allow the death of the white cells which normally live in small numbers in any organ, and these "passenger" leucocytes are major sources of immunogenicity. There are workers who believe that Summerlin genuinely was onto something, and that eventually his technique, though not valid for skin, may prove of value in transplanting endocrine glands such as the thyroid or pancreas. In any case, such organs appear to be less violently rejected than the kidney, heart, or liver.

In the case of diabetes, it may happen that the kidneys are destroyed by complications of the disease. The issue arises as to whether the patient should have a *combined* transplant of kidney and pancreas (certain cells of which manufacture insulin, and are malfunctioning in the diabetic). Certainly, if pancreas transplantation could be perfected without condemning the patient to a lifetime of immunosuppression, it would represent an interesting alternative to twice-daily injections of insulin going on for life. Still, the transplant barrier remains to plague us. The combined transplants, with a few notable exceptions, have not engendered much enthusiasm.

An undue amount of publicity has been given to a few physiological experiments in animals involving transplantation of the brain. Not even the most science-fiction-minded of transplantation biologists is thinking in terms of transplantation of the brain as a therapeutic procedure. To perform any useful function, the brain must have input and output. Otherwise it is like the idle central processing unit of a computer which is being fed no data and has been divorced from its printer. The millions of nerve fibers which serve as communication links between the sense organs and the brain, on the one hand, and the brain and the muscles, on the other, could not possibly be repaired by any process known or even remotely envisaged. Certainly a transplanted brain, given adequate oxygenation, will continue to be electrically active for some hours or days, and this may prove to be a useful tool in neurophysiological research. But the goal of preserving a great thinker's brain after death is still as firmly in the realm of fiction as it was when Roald Dahl described it so amusingly in *Kiss, Kiss*.

Transplantation of the lung in experimental animals has been disappointing. There are great technical problems, and postoperative pneumonia frequently occurs in the presence of immunosuppressive drugs. This is an area deserving of further work, but it will probably be one of the later avenues to be explored in man. The rejoining of severed limbs is not really a subject for this book. The questions are not immunological but surgical, and mainly involve the difficulty of obtaining an adequate nerve supply to and from the severed limb. A number of other organs and tissues will certainly also engage the attentions of the transplanters of the future.

Ethical, Legal, and Logistic Problems of Transplantation

There has been much controversy about the ethical and moral aspects of kidney transplantation using living volunteer donors. It is true that a person can get on quite well and live to a ripe old age with just one kidney. However, there is always the possibility that a kidney stone, infection, cancer or some other disease may change the remaining kidney. Also, the kidney could be injured in an accident. Finally, the donor is, after all, subjected to a major operation. All surgery carries some risk, and though no serious complications have yet arisen in any donor anywhere in the world, sooner or later there will be an anesthetic complication or a blood clot in the lungs which will put the donor in jeopardy. It seems to me that the propriety of using living donors depends largely on the difference in comparative success rates of programs using cadaver material versus living volunteer grafts. At the moment, this gap is not too wide, and may close further as genetic matching techniques improve. Living volunteers should certainly be seriously considered in the case of identical twins or MHC-identical siblings, but in most other circumstances, cadaver grafts are preferable. Matching procedures as applied to families bring with them a specially grave ethical problem. Suppose there are six children in a family. One contracts a fatal kidney disease and is in need of a graft. The other five children and the sick child have their white cells typed, and it turns out that only one of the five is a suitable donor. The psychological pressure under which that one donor is placed is so intense that some experts have wondered whether he is capable of exercising free will in the ordinary sense. On the other hand, experience so far has shown that relatives in general are only too ready to donate a kidney, even though they know that there is a substantial chance of rejection. The prob-

lem is a very knotty one and will best be solved when cadaver
grafts are so uniformly successful that the question of living
volunteer grafting hardly arises.

There are many medicolegal and logistic problems in both
living volunteer and cadaver transplant operations. The most
ideal source of cadaver organs would be accident victims, who
are usually healthy and often young. Still, there are big problems in getting the organ to a hospital sufficiently rapidly. While
some countries are now encouraging people to carry cards on
them authorizing organs to be taken for transplantation in case
of sudden death, the procedure is not yet very widespread and
it is more usual to obtain permission from relatives. These,
understandably, are in great distress and not easy to approach.
A common source of donor material is the patient who has had
a neurological accident such as a cerebral hemorrhage. In such
cases, the patient frequently goes into a prolonged coma before
dying. This gives some time during which the relatives become
accustomed to the possibility of death, and doctors can usually
find appropriate ways of asking for permission to remove a
kidney immediately after death. There is perhaps something
ghoulish in the thought that immediately after a person's death,
a whole tribe of surgeons may descend on the body ready to
remove kidneys, heart, liver, lungs, pancreas, and any other
bits and pieces that they can get hold of. This block is largely
in our minds. Most people in good health would agree that their
own organs would be better employed, after their death, in
helping to keep another person alive than in being burnt in a
crematorium or buried in a coffin.

As kidney grafts become more successful, logistic problems in
transplantation are developing. Suitable cadavers do not turn
up very frequently in a hospital. Moreover, blood group and
white-cell matching may indicate that the dying person is not
compatible with the various kidney graft patients in the hospital
at that time. There are difficulties in bringing adequate numbers
of potential organ donors and recipients together. These can be

overcome by careful community planning. Kidney sufferers can be kept alive almost indefinitely by repeated hemodialysis. There should be one center in each community adequately equipped to perform these dialyses on a waiting list of sick people. In this way, a pool of potential recipients of substantial size can build up. These patients would not be confined to hospitals. Over the waiting period, they would simply visit the kidney clinic twice per week for a stay of eight to twelve hours. A system could also be developed by which the same hospital could receive for care all seriously ill neurological cases; alternatively, deceased people could be brought very rapidly to the clinic concerned. Typing procedures would be carried out on hospital patients almost as routinely as blood typing, so the histocompatibility genotype of the donor would be known before death. When a particular donor actually dies or is about to die, the patient on the waiting list who most closely matches him is rushed to the hospital and grafting can take place as shortly after the death of the donor as possible.

This is the most sane and logical way for transplantation to develop. Cadaver transplants can harm no one, and can do untold good. We can end on much the same note as we started. Doctors can confer immortality on no one, and everyone has the right to die with dignity. Transplantation is now, and for the foreseeable future will remain, a last-ditch procedure to rescue a gravely ill person, too young to die, from what would otherwise be inevitable demise. Prevention and conventional treatment of kidney and other diseases will be far preferable to transplantation. The latter must be regarded as an adjunct to, and not a replacement for, standard medical practice. In this limited context, transplantation has already achieved much for the welfare of man. Its future can hardly fail to be even brighter than its spectacular recent past.

18

ALLERGY AND HYPERSENSITIVITY

O F ALL the many refined mechanisms that have been fashioned over the millennia by Darwinian evolution, antibody formation as seen in mammals is one of the most complex and delicate. In this chapter and the next we will be examining instances where antibody formation brings harm rather than good to the body. Here we are in an area where we can do little more than describe the phenomena and their treatment. For example, we cannot answer in any detailed way the obvious question of why some people are prone to allergies and others not. We suspect that genetic factors are the most important, but we do not know why evolution has allowed what to us seems a harmful tendency to become so common in the population. Frequently, while we can treat the symptoms, and have a deep understanding of the sequence of events that is occurring, we are frustratingly unable to come to grips with the fundamental flaw, the actual synthesis of harmful antibodies.

Allergy

At least 10 percent of people suffer from allergies of one sort or another. Allergy takes various forms, the most common being hay fever, hives, asthma, childhood eczema, and food allergies. Hay fever is an itchiness in the nose and eyes, with inflammation of the mucous membranes of the nose and sinuses, leading to sneezing and increased mucus secretion from the nose. Hives are itchy, raised lumps in the skin which come and go quickly and leave no marks. Asthma is a disorder in which there are attacks of difficulty in breathing owing to spasm in the passages that bring air to the lungs (the bronchial tubes). There is also increased mucous secretion in the bronchial tubes, and asthma sufferers frequently cough up thick sputum. Asthma is the most serious disease in this group, though fortunately it is often quite mild. Severe cases suffer a major handicap, though new inhalable drugs have greatly improved the outlook. Eczema is a skin rash, frequently particularly severe in the skin folds such as behind the knees or in front of the elbows. In severely affected children it can cover most of the body. Food allergies cause stomach cramps, hives, and other uncomfortable symptoms when certain foods (for example, strawberries, or shellfish) are eaten by susceptible people. The mechanisms of all of these have much in common and so frequently one person may suffer simultaneously or sequentially from a number of different allergies.

The tendency toward allergy is inherited and most allergic patients give a definite family history of some trouble. For example, if the patient has asthma, one brother may have hives, the father might suffer from hay fever, and two uncles and a cousin might all also be asthma sufferers. Such histories are common but not universal. The allergic patient may also give an interesting personal history. He may present for treatment of severe hay fever, and may give a history of childhood eczema, asthma in his teens which he has grown out of, and hay fever coming on in adult life. The severity of these allergic manifestations is very variable. Some people are so severely afflicted, particularly with asthma, that their health is seriously undermined and their life affected. Others have symptoms that are so trivial that they do not even consult a doctor, and there are all stages in between.

The central causative agent in allergies is an antibody. Allergic patients make antibodies of a special kind to a variety of weakly antigenic substances called *allergens*, whereas normal people make these antibodies in only trace amounts. Allergic antibodies are called *reagins*, and belong to the IgE class of immunoglobulins. The special property of reaginic antibodies is to fix onto cells in skin and mucous surfaces called mast cells. The first time a person meets an allergen no harm results but formation of reagins starts. Typical allergens include assorted pollens, components of household dust, various feathers, and certain foods. In each case, the antigen is one which enters the body not by injection or infection, but by making contact with some inner or outer body lining. In most instances, the detailed chemical nature of the antigen is not known, though this is not true for some common allergens such as ragweed pollen found in North America. Most people do not respond when exposed to ingested or inhaled allergens. More than 10 percent of people do, at least to some of them, and form the reaginic antibody. This is made in specialized collections of lymphoid tissue beneath the lining of the respiratory or gastrointestinal tract. The IgE, once formed, attaches to the mast cell which has a special receptor for IgE on its surface. The union is quite firm and stable. When the person meets the allergen for the second time, a sequence of events occurs, as shown in Figure 18–1. The antigenic determinants of the allergen (which has to be at least bivalent) cross-link two or more IgE molecules. This causes the relevant receptors to aggregate much as in the case of Ig mole-

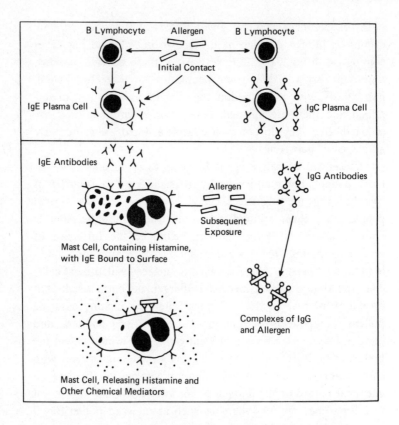

Figure 18–1. Cellular phenomena in allergy. Initially, contact of an allergen with the lymphoid system leads to antibody production. As well as the normal IgG antibodies, IgE antibodies are formed. The latter attach to mast cells, and a later exposure to the same allergen can cause aggregation of the surface IgE molecules and a release of mast cell granules, liberating histamine and other inflammatory substances. The IgG antibody may have a "blocking" role, mopping up the allergen and preventing it getting to the mast cell. However, IgG-antigen complexes may have a variety of irritating effects in the body.

cules on the B cell surface when "patched" and "capped" by
anti-Ig (Chapter 13). The result appears to be the creation of
a calcium pore, and calcium ions rush into the cell. This causes
preformed granules inside the mast cell to rupture and release
their contents, including two powerful pharmacologically active
agents, histamine and heparin. Histamine acts powerfully on
small blood vessels, causing them to dilate and allow the seep-
age out of excessive amounts of fluid. It also acts on the
muscles inside bronchial tubes, in which it causes a constriction.
Other powerful chemicals are also synthesized and/or released
following antigen-antibody union. They include serotonin, slow-
reacting substance A, and eosinophil chemotactic factor A.
These other chemicals are also powerful substances in inflammation. Why the union of antigen and antibodies in tissues
should have such drastic effects is a mystery. Presumably it
reflects in some way the fact that if the antigen had been a
harmful bacterium, increased inflammation in the area might
have been a helpful factor in limiting its spread and bringing
extra granulocytes and monocytes to help fight it. Reaginic
antibody seems to be some kind of perversion of this useful
function.

We will not discuss extensively the treatment of allergies, but
this can be divided into two broad types. First, there are drugs
which suppress the symptoms. Second, there are desensitization
procedures, the aim of which is to prevent the harmful antigen-
antibody union. The drugs used are chosen in order to counter-
act the pharmacological agents which have been released by
the body itself. The effects of histamine release are fought by
the common and well-known antihistaminic drugs. These do not
inhibit histamine release but help to prevent inflammation by
competing with histamine for receptors on smooth muscle and
capillaries. Taken one to three times per day in pill form, they
are helpful in controlling the milder manifestations of allergies.
For severe disturbances they can be given by injection. Another
group of drugs, especially helpful in asthma, in that which

counteracts the vessel dilatation and bronchial spasm by mimicking the action of the sympathetic nerves, those going to blood vessels and muscles. Drugs in this group, which cause small vessels to contract and the bronchial tubes to relax, are called sympathomimetic agents, and include adrenaline and many related compounds. Again, mild symptoms can be relieved by drugs taken in tablet form or inhaled as an aerosol, but severe ones may require injections. Finally, in very severe allergies, it may be necessary to invoke the powerful anti-inflammatory properties of the cortisone group of drugs.

Desensitization represents another approach to the allergy problem. It consists, not of treating a particular attack, but of attempts to prevent the union of antigen with antibodies. First, the allergist must find out to what substance a person is allergic. To do this, he takes a careful history to see if the patient can pin down the attacks to any particular exposure, such as to going out in the garden in springtime, sweeping the floor, sleeping on a feather pillow, and so forth. This may give a clue as to the probable nature of the allergen. The next step is a series of skin tests. The materials to which the patient may be allergic are applied to the skin in one of a variety of ways which ensure some permeation into the deeper layers. If the patient is allergic to something, an area of redness and swelling will appear in the skin owing to histamine release. This procedure is uncomfortable, and may rarely be dangerous. It is increasingly being replaced by laboratory tests on the patient's serum which determine the presence and amount of IgE antibodies to particular allergens. Once the allergens have been identified, the allergist must decide whether to proceed with desensitization. Frequently, the patient is allergic to so many different things at once that it is not practicable even to attempt desensitization. However, if there seems to be one, or at least a predominant, allergen, desensitization can be attempted. This consists essentially of a course of injections of the allergen. At first, very small amounts are used, and then progressively larger amounts are given. Injections are given several times per week, and a course lasts for several months. The rationale that is most frequently given is that the injections cause the formation of "blocking antibodies." These are believed to be non-skin-fixing antibodies which are supposed to compete with the reagins for the allergen. They are supposed to combine with the allergen and "mop it up" before the reagin fixed to cells can unite with it. Another idea about desensitization which has been put forward recently is that the series of injections induces not immunity but tolerance. The many injections may cause a progressive diminution of reagin synthesis. There is still considerable controversy over the real value of desensitization courses. Many individual patients with hay fever do seem to get real benefit, but in most fully controlled "double-blind" trials of injection treatment in asthma, where neither the patient nor the doctor know whether the injections contained allergen or simply distilled water, the differences between the benefit obtained in treated and control patients have been rather marginal. It is to be hoped that with the continued progress in immunological knowledge, desensitization procedures may be placed on a progressively sounder footing.

Serum Sickness and Related Phenomena

Soluble complexes of antigen and antibody can be very injurious to a variety of body tissues. A good example is the reaction that some people develop to injections of horse serum. When people are injured in an accident, doctors frequently used to inject a small amount of passive antibody against tetanus, prepared by immunizing a horse, in order to prevent even a remote possibility of this disease. In a number of individuals, the second or subsequent time that the horse proteins are injected a variety of symptoms may occur, collectively termed accelerated serum disease. These include hives, skin rashes, bronchial spasm, lowering of the blood pressure, shock, and occasionally even death. These follow immediately on injection into the individual who has been pre-immunized by the previous injection. The cause of these adverse reactions is again related to antigen-antibody union. The initial injection of horse serum has caused antibody formation. Soluble complexes of antigen and antibody form rapidly after the second injection and can have severe direct irritating effects on tissues. They can also cause complement fixation and a variety of other deleterious chain reactions. Particularly violent reactions are induced when the horse serum or other antigen is injected directly into a vein. In the severest instances, the result can be acute anaphylaxis, a severe state of shock which can lead to death in minutes. Fortunately it is unusual for people to form substantial amounts of antibody to horse serum after a small number of injections, and severe forms of anaphylactic shock are quite rare. Nevertheless, the routine use of horse anti-tetanus serum has now been abandoned, as it does more harm than good in the long run. A much better approach is to achieve nationwide immunization against tetanus during childhood and give a booster injection of active immunization at the time of a cut or other accident. If, for some reason, the victim has not been immunized before, combined immunization with tetanus toxoid and a prophylactic course of antibiotics will provide protection against tetanus. In some instances, where a wound is deep and dirty, and it is felt that tetanus antiserum must be given, then human material is preferable. This is now available in many countries.

Sometimes the first administration of foreign serum can cause *serum sickness*. This is not immediate but occurs some 10 days or so after the passive antibody shot. The symptoms consist of fever, swollen joints, skin rashes, and kidney problems, all of which usually resolve within some days. Serum sickness arises in the following way: the antigen, horse serum, is given and causes antibody formation after a period of seven to ten days. At that time, there may still be antigen molecules present in the circulation. Antigen and antibody unite, complexes are formed, and they irritate many tissues.

Another example of hypersensitivity, and a very serious one, is drug hypersensitivity. A small proportion of people given penicillin will form IgE antibody to it, or more frequently to traces of related compounds present in penicillin preparations. A subsequent injection of penicillin in such a sensitized individual can give rise to any one of the many symptoms described above. Anything from acute anaphylactic shock to merely a skin rash may result. Fortunately, severe penicillin hypersensitivity is rare, but it does represent the most serious complication of this marvelous drug. There are numerous drugs which exceptionally give rise to immunological complications, by a variety of quite different mechanisms. Occasionally these can take a bizarre form, such as the bleeding tendency which may occur when drug-IgG-antibody complexes hook onto blood platelets and cause complement fixation and platelet destruction. Platelets are little pieces of cytoplasm which float in the blood and are vital to the clotting mechanism. When they are destroyed, a gross bleeding tendency develops. The field of drug hypersensitivity is fascinating and complex. The presence of these types of unwanted side effects of drugs is one of the reasons why it is never wise to take any form of drug without medical supervision.

Delayed Hypersensitivity

In Chapter 4, we encountered delayed hypersensitivity as a laboratory phenomenon, where immunized T cells initiated an inflammatory cascade after introduction of an antigen into the skin. Unfortunately, the same series of events can occur in nature. Frequently what happens is that a chemical is absorbed through the skin, for example through occupational exposure. The chemical attaches to some self-protein, the conjugate is immunogenic, and T lymphocytes reactive against the chemical are formed. The next exposure to the antigen elicits an angry, delayed rash similar to a whole series of tuberculin reactions. This so-called "contact sensitivity" frequently enters a chronic phase, resulting in a scaly, itchy, distressing rash. Contact sensitivity is very difficult to treat, and one must identify the antigen at fault and remove the patient from contact with it, even if this means changing occupation. Sensitivity to cosmetics is a common variant of contact sensitivity.

This description of the more common allergies and hypersensitivities is by no means exhaustive, and it would not have been difficult to fill a whole book on the present subject. What is rather upsetting is that the incredible mass of detailed information about IgE, mast cells, T cell regulation of IgE responses, immunological tolerance, suppressor T cells, and many related topics, even since the first edition of *Antibodies and Immunity*, has not yet led to a better deal for the allergic patient. Many hopeful leads appear on the horizon. One fascinating one, already in extensive clinical use, is a drug, taken by inhalation, which specifically inhibits mast cell degranulation. Allergists as a group are learning more imunology, and are thus getting progressively more ready to tackle the problem logically rather than empirically.

19

AUTOIMMUNITY

I N OUR STUDY of allergy, we saw how things can go wrong when cells make antibodies against certain foreign antigens. In many cases, trouble can be averted simply by avoiding contact with the relevant antigen. The hay fever sufferer may stay indoors in springtime. The person sensitive to penicillin will make sure that no doctor prescribes the drug for him again. We will now turn to an examination of a malfunctioning of the immune system where such escape is not possible. We have mentioned that Paul Ehrlich coined the phrase "horror auto-toxicus," which describes vividly his picture of the horror and chaos which could result if the lymphocytes started to mount an immune attack against autologous constituents. This would represent a form of civil warfare—white cells against red, lymphocytes against liver and kidney—leading to anarchy and to grave disease. In fact, a limited form of such civil warfare is not uncommon and the diseases in which it occurs are called autoimmune diseases. Sometimes, indeed, these are life-threatening, but many are milder than you might imagine. The original prototypes of autoimmune diseases were rather rare conditions—"small print stuff" as far as general practitioners and medical students are concerned. However, as more clinical researchers began to look for autoantibodies, a greater number of diseases were found in which antibodies made by the person against the diseased organ were a prominent part of the overall picture. Autoimmunity is now a topical concept and relevant to many common diseases.

The advancing front of science is usually characterized by an atmosphere of spirited controversy. Research is at its most exciting when full interpretations of all the relevant facts are not yet at hand. This is the stage when there is room for critical analysis, imagination, and creative theorizing. Immunology, from the days of Metchnikoff onward, has been full of such controversies, and the field of autoimmunity is no exception. On the one hand, some experts have proposed that aggressive lymphocytes and autoantibodies are actually the causes of the diseases. The tendency to form autoantibodies is believed to represent an intrinsically sick lymphoid system which is responding abnormally to autologous constituents. The chief proponents of this view have been Sir Macfarlane Burnet and Dr. I. R. Mackay from The Walter and Eliza Hall Institute in Melbourne, and the late Dr. William Dameshek of Boston. They have coined the phrase "forbidden clone" to describe the proliferating lymphoid cells responsible for tissue damage. The concept covers both antibody-forming cells and lymphocytes which inflict target cell damage by a direct cellular immune attack. An alternate view, which has many adherents among American medical scientists, is that the real, basic cause of diseases characterized by autoantibodies is still unknown. This unknown cause induces tissue damage. As a result, many kinds of molecules are released from the damaged tissue. These may include molecules which are normally not present in significant concentration in the circulation, and so the body has had no chance to become tolerant to them. According to this alternate concept, the release of these previously sequestered antigens is followed by a normal immune response mounted by normal lymphoid cells.

The autoantibodies and aggressive lymphocytes are merely an index of tissue damage, and not its root cause. The view has been expressed that the fundamental cause may be some form of unusual virus, but no experimental proof of this has been given. Several compromise solutions have also been proposed. For example, some people may be genetically more disposed than others to respond to the triggering stimulus of a transient appearance of autoantigens. Also, it is possible that the original antigen release, cause unknown, is followed by a vicious cycle. Thus, tissue damage causes antigen release which causes an immune response which causes more tissue damage and more antigen release. Such a cycle could explain many features of autoimmunity.

Whatever the initiating cause, there is no doubt that autoantibodies can do very severe harm. Consideration of just one autoimmune condition, called hemolytic anemia, makes this quite clear. In this disease, the patient makes antibodies against his own red blood cells which cause their destruction, leading to a severe and sometimes fatal anemia. Here, the idea that the antibody is simply an index of tissue damage clearly does not hold water. In other situations, the correlation between lymphocyte and plasma cell infiltration of an organ, followed by progressive decline in function, is so strong that it is impossible to escape a cause-and-effect conclusion. The validity of autoimmunity as a mechanism for disease is further strengthened by certain laboratory-induced conditions, which we will consider below.

Since the first edition of *Antibodies and Immunity*, the virus theory has gained ground as a result of observations in mice, chickens, and mink; but no clear-cut example of a human autoimmune disease-associated virus exists except for the transient appearance of autoantibodies in the self-limited disease, glandular fever. On the other hand, the forbidden clone notion has also received some support from the discovery that suppressor T cells are important in controlling B cell function. The idea that autoimmunity results from deficiency in suppressor T cells, failing in their job of controlling autoantibody formation, gains support from some authors.

It is probably wrong to attempt to squeeze all of the diverse phenomena within autoimmunity into a single causative heading. When the field is more completely understood, it may well be that all the above views can find a place in the total picture. It remains by way of introduction to mention the vital role of genetics (Chapter 15). Clearly some autoimmune processes occur only in the presence of the "right" immune response genes.

Experimental Autoimmune Disease

If one takes perfectly normal, adult laboratory animals and injects into them extracts of certain tissues, one can cause the production of diseases similar in many respects to human auto-immune disorders. For example, one can remove one-half of a rabbit's thyroid, a ductless or endocrine gland situated in the neck, grind up the tissue and inject it back into the same rabbit together with an adjuvant which heightens the immune response. The remaining half-thyroid develops a chronic inflammation leading to thyroid deficiency. Antithyroid antibodies appear in the serum and histological sections of the gland reveal an infil- tration with lymphocytes very reminiscent of that seen in human autoimmune thyroiditis. Other experimental autoimmune dis- eases that have been extensively studied and have human parallels include encephalitis (brain inflammation), produced by injection of brain antigens in adjuvants, and adrenalitis (adrenal disease), induced in a basically similar manner. While these experimental conditions resemble their counterparts in human clinical medicine to a degree, they differ in a number of respects. Human autoimmune diseases tend to go on for long periods of time, being sometimes a little better, sometimes worse, but really coming to an end only when the organ being attacked has been entirely destroyed. Experimental autoimmune conditions are rarely as persistent as this. Usually there is an acute phase which ends in either the death of the animal or a spontaneous cure. The vicious cycle type of natural history is not usually found. Furthermore, while some human autoimmune conditions affect a multiplicity of organs and tissues, experimental autoimmune disease usually affects only those organs from which the antigens used to induce the disease were derived.

Examples of Human Autoimmune Diseases

One useful way of classifying human autoimmune diseases is into two major groups: those in which predominantly one organ is affected, and those in which the disease process is diffused through many tissues. Let us consider key examples of the first group. An important one is acquired *hemolytic anemia*. This is a disease in which the patient makes antibodies to his own red cells. Normal red cells live for about a hundred days in man; red cells attacked by antibodies live for only a few days. In hemolytic anemia there is therefore grossly excessive red blood cell destruction. Most red cells are destroyed in the spleen, and in this disease the spleen has so much work to do that it becomes greatly enlarged and swollen. This enlargement can be felt by the doctor when he examines the abdomen and can be an important clue to the diagnosis. Final proof comes from laboratory tests which show that the patient's red cells are coated with antibodies. The colored pigments in red cells (which make them red) are released in excessive amount as the spleen destroys the cells. Various enzymes convert them into yellowish pigments which can give these patients a jaundiced appearance. These are finally excreted in the bile. If the liver, which makes bile, is perfectly healthy, the jaundice of these patients will not be as deep or persistent as that in certain forms of liver or bile duct disease. Though the bone marrow tries hard to make up for the excess destruction by pouring out new red cells, it can never quite catch up and anemia develops. We will deal in general with the treatment of autoimmune diseases shortly, but in this particular disease the condition can frequently be considerably improved by removing the spleen. This allows the antibody-coated red cells to live and function longer, with a resulting higher level of red cells in the blood.

Another good example of this first group of diseases is chronic thyroiditis, sometimes called Hashimoto's disease, after the Japanese doctor who first described it. This involves a slow deterioration of the thyroid, which finally results in its complete destruction and replacement by fibrous tissue. Fortunately, the patient can be restored to excellent health simply by taking thyroid tablets to replace the lost function. Pernicious anemia is a common disease which also belongs in this group. This is a condition caused by defective absorption of certain vitamins, particularly vitamin B_{12}, from the stomach wall. The mucous lining of the stomach becomes chronically inflamed and finally the specialized cells are destroyed altogether. Special factors necessary for vitamin B_{12} absorption cannot then be made. More recently, the interesting notion has come up that some autoimmune diseases are due to antibodies and/or cytotoxic T cells to specialized receptors on cell membranes. For example, a severe disease called myasthenia gravis (serious muscle weakness) may be due to an autoimmune attack against the receptor at the nerve-muscle junction, which normally has the job of welcoming the chemical neurotransmitter molecule, acetyl choline.

The second group of autoimmune diseases is best exemplified by one with a long name: *systemic lupus erythematosus* (SLE).

This is a condition affecting the skin, joints, lymph nodes and spleen, liver, lung, gastrointestinal tract, and, above all, the kidneys. Progressive destructive change in the kidneys is the commonest cause of death in SLE. A good proportion of the damage in the various organs can be ascribed, not so much to a direct antibody attack on the organs, but to the irritating effects of antigen-antibody complexes. In this disease, antibodies to the person's own DNA and to various other constituents of cell nuclei are formed. These antibodies react with the nuclei of lymphocytes present in the circulation, and also with various digestive breakdown products of cell nuclei. Many types of antigen-antibody complexes form and exert a variety of irritant effects. For example, in the kidney they sludge out of the circulation and form dense deposits which interfere with the correct filtration of urine. The deposits of antigen-antibody complexes cause changes which are easy to spot on electron-microscopic sections. You will see that SLE has features in common with serum sickness, a form of hypersensitivity discussed in the preceding chapter. In serum sickness, the antigen is quickly eliminated and the disease self-limited. In SLE, the antigens are universal and ever-present. The patient will usually suffer from the disease to a greater or lesser degree for the rest of life, though with good treatment SLE patients can now survive for many years.

How can we tell that a particular disorder is autoimmune in nature? This is not easy, even for specialists in internal medicine. There are five markers of autoimmunity that have been suggested as useful guides by Mackay and Burnet. First, auto-antibodies to one or more types of tissue are present. Second, the total amount of immunoglobulin in the serum is usually well above normal limits. Third, accumulations of lymphocytes and plasma cells occur in the affected tissues. Fourth, the patient receives significant benefit from being treated with cortisone or an equivalent immunosuppressive drug. Finally, more than one manifestation of autoimmunity may occur in the patient, and a family history of autoimmune symptoms and signs is common. Many autoimmune patients exhibit all five markers, and a confident diagnosis can usually be made if the first and three of the other four are present.

Moving from established facts onto more speculative ground, we can consider briefly some very important diseases that cannot yet be classified as autoimmune but might with further research come into the camp. One candidate is diabetes, one of the most common of all severe diseases, which afflicts about one in fifty of all people in Western communities. Diabetes is not just one disease. It comes in two main forms. The first, juvenile diabetes, begins at a young age, is more severe, invariably requires insulin, and can be dangerously unstable and followed by serious complications. The second, mature onset diabetes, is milder overall and may sometimes be controlled by diet alone. Research workers have long striven to ascribe the former type, where insulin fails to be produced, to autoimmune destruction of the insulin-producing cells of the pancreas. This is particularly the case as so many disturbances of other endocrine glands, including the thyroid, adrenal, and ovary, are now known to be autoimmune. The trouble has been that, though anti-pancreatic cell antibodies have occasionally been noted, large numbers of diabetics have not shown an impressively high incidence of autoantibodies. The reason for this has recently emerged. It appears that autoimmune antibodies appear very early in the disease, wreak their havoc, and disappear again. When a randomly chosen group of diabetics is taken, there will be a few cases of recent onset with autoantibodies, but most cases of longer established duration are usually antibody-negative. Once again, as in all the above examples, it is possible that much of the damage is due not to the autoantibodies as such but to auto-aggressive killer T cells concomitantly present.

Now that medical researchers are fully alerted to the existence of immune mechanisms of tissue damage, there is no telling how widely the net may finally be cast. For example, some recent authors have even been courageous enough to suggest that hypertension and coronary artery disease may be partly caused by immune mechanisms. While few would speculate that far, the field of immunopathology has made great strides in its quarter-century old history.

Genetic Factors in Human Autoimmunity

The classical autoimmune diseases are rare, and a straight-forward family history, such as is frequently observed in allergies, is not usual. However, genetic factors are nevertheless very important. The most clear-cut is the dependence of some autoimmune diseases on some MHC alleles. It is also evident that relatives of patients with an autoimmune disease show low levels of the relevant (or a related) autoantibody more frequently than does a random population. The innate tendency is there, but is held in check. Furthermore, family trees may show that a relative suffered from a *related* disorder. The patient may have pernicious anemia; the mother or aunt might have autoimmune thyroid disease. Analysis suggests not a simple hereditary mechanism such as in hemophilia, but rather an inheritance based on mutiple gene loci. Work in mice suggests that at least two gene sets are involved, one MHC-linked and one not.

If deficiency in suppressor T cells is really an important aspect of autoimmunity, it may help to explain the prevalence of autoantibodies in old age. A group of people sampled in a home for the aged will show a much higher incidence of autoantibodies than a group of young adults. Frequently, these cause no evident disease, modest levels of autoantibody formation being quite compatible with health. The thymus atrophies in old age, and there may well be a deficit in suppressor T cells and a partial breakdown of self-tolerance. The fact that the effects on the body are not more disastrous strongly suggests that suppressor T cells are only *one* of the mechanisms for self-tolerance, and clonal abortion (Chapter 12) may well underlie the absence of massive autoimmunity.

An interesting sidelight on some autoimmune diseases and also some allergies is a certain relationship to psychological stress. The psychological overtones in asthma are widely known, and several studies have claimed that a severe stress can precipitate an exacerbation or even the onset of autoimmune disease. Unfortunately, our capacity to quantitate psychological stress, and thus to study such concepts objectively, is limited. However, it is by no means farfetched to incriminate the brain and nervous system in immune phenomena. The nervous system controls the hypothalamus, which controls the pituitary, which in turn controls all the endocrine glands. The balance of hormones is certainly important in relation to the thymus and lymphocyte levels, not to speak of the effects of blood flow on the health of tissues and perhaps on antigen leakage from them. This research field, just starting to gain a degree of respectability, is clearly important for the future of medicine.

Genetic Factors in Autoimmunity Occurring Spontaneously in Mice

Apart from the autoimmune conditions induced artificially in experimental animals by intentional injections of autoantigens in Freund's adjuvant, there is another and even more important type of autoimmunity which can be investigated in the laboratory. There are certain inbred strains of mice which, spontaneously and without any interference by the investigator, develop autoimmune diseases. These strains were discovered by a group of New Zealand geneticists and are called by the initials NZ, plus an initial describing the coat color; thus, NZB for New Zealand black, NZW for New Zealand white mice, and so forth. These mice really do seem to have an inherited proneness for a variety of conditions similar to the human diseases which we have been considering. Practically all of the NZB mice develop hemolytic anemia, with gross enlargement of the spleen. A hybrid between NZB and NZW develops a disease very like human SLE. Female mice quite uniformly develop severe SLE kidney disease, and without treatment 100 percent are dead by one year of age. This corresponds to age thirty-five in a human. These extraordinary mouse strains have contributed to our knowledge of autoimmunity in three major ways. First, because the mice are strictly inbred, a detailed study of the influence of genetic factors in disease incidence has been made possible. Second, because of the predictable nature of the disease process, it is possible to study pathological mechanisms before symptoms actually occur; in other words, it is as though a human patient walked into the clinic several years before he became ill and said: "I will develop SLE in seven years. Do something about it!" Third, because the disease is in an experimental animal and not in a person, a much more extensive series of investigations and trial treatments can be performed than would be ethical in a human.

While genetic factors (probably at least two sets of genes) are vitally important, viruses also play a part in NZ mouse disease. In the case of the SLE-like disease, it is clear that much of the disastrous immune complex formation involves antibodies to a common mouse virus particle. These so-called C-type particles occur in many mouse strains and may themselves do no harm, but antibodies against them lead to immune complex formation and kidney disease. Again, this may represent failure of suppressor T cells to limit antibody formation against a persisting antigen.

Studies of NZ mice that are not yet sick have also been

revealing. Young NZB mice that are still perfectly healthy already show certain abnormalities that are probably correlated with the later development of hemolytic anemia. For example, they have excessive levels of IgM globulin in their serum, and they show an abnormal thymic architecture. NZB/NZW hybrids can be seen to have microscopic areas of damage in their kidneys long before they actually become sick. An analysis of this injury led to the conclusion that the damage was due, at least in part, to antigen-antibody complexes. Sequential autopsies of mice killed before they would have become sick, and at intervals during the various stages of the disease, have given us deep insights into the way in which things get progressively worse in these conditions if untreated, and have materially helped our understanding of the human counterparts. Most important of all, studies of NZ mice have shown that it is more difficult than in other strains to induce immunological tolerance to test antigens in them, and to generate effective suppressor T cells. This could well be the key genetic defect underlying their many problems.

Best of all is the opportunity that the mouse models give us for trying out new drugs of possible use in treatment. For example, the kidney disease of NZB/NZW hybrids has been found to respond brilliantly to a drug called cyclophosphamide. In the mice, even relatively brief courses of treatment arrest the kidney disease. Longer-term treatment allows the mice to live to a healthy old age—about double their untreated life span. The mice are clearly a gold mine in any further search for new therapeutic agents. Of course, the leap from mouse to man cannot be made abruptly. The species differ, the diseases are alike but not identical, the way each animal processes, degrades, and excretes drugs will vary. But patient and intelligent work in the mouse will surely be rewarded by the eventual development of better forms of treatment for man.

Autoimmunity and Lymphoid Malignancy

Proponents of the "forbidden clone" origin of autoimmune disease have drawn attention to an interesting finding which, they feel, supports the notion that it is basically the lymphoid cells that are at fault in these disorders. No one can dispute that leukemia, a malignant overgrowth of white cells, is basically a disease of these cells and their precursors. In leukemia, it is generally only one of the different types of white cells which is manufactured in gross excess. When the lymphocytes are involved, we have lymphatic leukemia. The observation relevant to this chapter is that patients with lymphatic leukemia frequently suffer from episodes of severe autoimmune attack. For example, sudden bouts of hemolytic anemia may complicate a case which is otherwise responding well to treatment. The fact that this will happen in 10 to 15 percent of patients indicates that this is not simply a coincidence of two unrelated disorders. The argument has been put forward by Dameshek that both leukemia and autoimmunity are "immunoproliferative disorders" in which abnormal cell division and abnormal cell function go hand in hand. Autoimmune manifestations also occur in other basically immunological diseases including those called lymphosarcoma, macroglobulinemia, and agammaglobulinemia. The fact that autoimmunity is so common in lymphocytic disorders argues strongly against the notion that autoimmunity is always caused by release of sequestered antigens.

Treatment of Autoimmune Disease

The treatment of autoimmune diseases in man revolves around three themes: first, to reduce the intensity of the immunological damage; second, to replace any vital bodily function that has been rendered defective through tissue destruction; third, to give general supportive and symptomatic treatment. Under the first heading, we include drugs that we have already discussed in Chapter 17. In fact, the treatment of autoimmunity has much in common with the treatment of graft rejection episodes; both are associated with the aggressive action of lymphocytes, and in both cases proliferation is necessary to build up the army of destroyers. In both cases, the chief drugs used are cortisone-like agents and cell-multiplication poisons. In grafts a combination of the two types of drugs is standard treatment. In many autoimmune diseases the same is now the case, though details of treatment vary considerably from disease to disease. For example, in many instances, it may be preferable to limit one's treatment to a replacement of the hormone no longer made because of autoimmune destruction of endocrine tissue. This second major approach to therapy is exemplified by treatment of thyroid autoimmunity by thyroid tablets or pernicious anemia by Vitamin B_{12}. It happens that some autoimmune diseases burn themselves out, frequently because of total destruction of the tissue at risk. There is then no point whatever in attempting to repel the aggressors with powerful, dangerous drugs. There are occasions in which the first and second approaches must be used simultaneously; for example, in severe hemolytic anemia cortisone would be given, but specific measures aimed at rapidly making up for the red cell destruction would also be needed. This is accomplished by removing the spleen by surgery, which eliminates the chief site of red cell breakdown, and by giving blood transfusions, which must, however, be used sparingly, as the transferred red cells will also be subjected to antibody attack. The third line of treatment is logical and common to the whole of clinical medicine. At times doctors find themselves powerless to eliminate the root of the evil, but they can nevertheless give the patient a great deal of help in relieving pain, minimizing complications, and generally helping a person to live with the disease.

Though in many cases a complete cure of autoimmune disease is not achieved, it has been heartening to note what excellent and long lives many patients can lead while on maintenance doses of immunosuppressants. For example, in autoimmune liver disease, we make it a practice after three years of continuous treatment, usually with both prednisone and azathioprine, gradually to diminish and then withdraw the drugs. At the slightest biochemical evidence of relapse (which is frequent) drugs are reinstituted, but a proportion of patients do not require this. Most of the others continue to live normal lives, working and even bearing children. It is a far cry from the times when many of these conditions were considered a death sentence. This is not to say that we can afford to rest content with immunosuppression. As in the case of organ grafts, it represents a blunt weapon, and we must continue to strive to understand the causes and eradicate the roots of autoimmunity.

20

CANCER

CANCER is undoubtedly the most emotion-laden problem in medicine today. Not only is cancer still a major killer, second only to heart and arterial diseases as a cause of mortality in developed countries. It is also the cause of morbid and even exaggerated fears, which can delay reporting of symptoms and thus militate against early diagnosis and cure. But it is important to stress that many early cancers can be cured, and even in the field of advanced, metastatic cancer, rays of hope are beginning to appear. In particular, while no responsible investigator would claim that the immunological approach to cancer will soon provide a universal panacea, a large segment of cancer research today is concerned with the possibility of harnessing the body's immune defense system in the fight against cancer, and many useful experimental and clinical leads have emerged.

Benign and Malignant Tumors

A tumor, or neoplasm, is an overgrowth of tissue beyond the normal limits of size or healthy functioning. Tumors must be distinguished from the normal growth of tissues in response to physiological stimuli, such as the calluses on a gardener's hands or the bulging muscles of a weightlifter. There is fair room for variation in organ size. Tumors represent the growth of tissue outside this range.

By no means do all tumors represent serious hazards. Technically we divide tumors into *benign* and *malignant*. Benign tumors, as the name implies, grow relatively slowly. They do not grossly invade the surrounding tissues or diffuse widely through the body. A good example of a benign tumor is an ordinary mole; another, the round, fatty lumps that quite a few people have on their backs or elsewhere, which are called lipomas. If a benign tumor is externally situated it has at worst a cosmetically harmful effect. However, benign tumors in internal organs can be quite serious and even fatal. For example, a benign tumor in the brain can grow ever so slowly, causing no symptoms at all until it begins to press on vital nerve centers. If surgery is then undertaken, a complete cure can result, but if the case is left untreated, the patient may eventually die. Other benign tumors can harm the body by pouring out vast quantities of some hormone or metabolite, as can happen with pituitary or adrenal tumors.

Benign tumors frequently reach a definitive size and then stop growing. The essential feature of a malignant tumor or cancer is progressive growth. As the tumor mass enlarges, it invades surrounding tissues. Most but not all malignant tumors also possess the characteristic of spreading from the original site of origin of the tumor, via the lymphatic vessels and lymph nodes, and/or via the bloodstream. Cells are shed from the primary tumor mass and grow into satellite areas of tumor tissue in the new host organ. These secondary areas of cancer growth are called *metastases*, or, more loosely, secondaries.

Cancer can attack any organ or tissue and within a particular organ can display a variety of detailed histological appearances and growth characteristics. Over the centuries, an enormous amount of information has built up about the natural history of these many malignant tumors, their responses to surgery and other treatments, and their prognosis. Some cancers are much commoner than others. At the moment, the most frequent malignancies include cancer of the lung, large intestine, prostate, and stomach in men; and of the breast, uterus, ovaries, lung, and stomach in women, as well as various cancers of the white blood cell system (leukemias and lymphomas) in both sexes.

The Causes of Cancer

Cancer is certainly not a single disease, but rather a blanket term describing a large number of different and perhaps causally unrelated conditions. Moreover, it is clear in many instances that the induction of a cancer in a tissue is not a single event, but rather a multistage progression, with certain precancerous changes preceding the onset of malignancy, perhaps by years. Our knowledge of the causes of cancer comes chiefly from two sources. First, there are epidemiological studies in man. Thus, certain cancers occur in particular occupational groups (bladder cancer in aniline dye workers); individuals with particular habits (smoking and lung cancer); populations sharing defined risks (leukemia in the survivors of Hiroshima and Nagasaki); ethnic groups exhibiting common racial characteristics and cultural patterns (high stomach cancer rates in the Japanese); and so forth. This approach of epidemiology and geographical pathology in man has been crucially important in identifying *risk factors* in cancer induction. It cannot, of course, illuminate the sequence of pathological mechanisms occurring in cells and tissues. For this we must turn to the second large area of research, intentional induction of malignancy in experimental animals (frequently mice) or in cells placed in tissue culture. While this second approach has been important in enlarging our understanding of cancer causation, a cautionary note must be sounded. In nature, the latent period for cancer can be very long (e.g., thirty years of smoking), but in the laboratory the investigator prefers, or at times is forced, to develop models which induce cancer very powerfully and very quickly. These models may represent an exaggerated version of what really happens in man. The two approaches together have led to our present understanding of carcinogenesis. This can conveniently be discussed under the headings to follow.

Chemical Carcinogenesis

It has long been known that certain chemical substances can be carcinogenic. By now, there are hundreds of known chemical carcinogens, each with its own spectrum of tissue susceptibility, species pattern and dosage, and time requirements. In many models of chemical carcinogenesis, a combination of the chemical substance and mechanical irritation is required, the chemical representing the carcinogen, the irritant a co-carcinogen. Two classical examples are the cancer of the scrotum that used to be frequent among chimney sweeps, and the cancer of the lip among certain tribes of American Indians that smoked and chewed on pipes with a clay stem, often broken and jagged. In the laboratory much work has been done on painting carcinogenic hydrocarbons, such as methylcholanthrene, onto the skin of mice, together with croton oil, an irritant. A similar type of procedure involves injecting paraffin oil into the abdominal cavity of certain strains of mice. Some paraffin oils contain traces of carcinogens, which can be isolated and purified. All paraffins are intensely irritating to the lining of the abdomen, and cause the outpouring of a fluid exudate which contains many white cells. In the right genetic strain, a malignancy of plasma cells, termed multiple myeloma, results six to nine months after the injection. In other models of chemical carcinogenesis, no co-carcinogen is necessary. For example, the intravenous injection of dimethylnitrosamine into the rat causes tumors in many organs, particularly the kidney.

Scientists have been searching for a common feature in the action of chemical carcinogens on cells, and one has now been found. It appears that all carcinogens either are themselves mutagenic or are converted by the body into a mutagen. A mutagen is a substance or agent that increases the rate of mutation in dividing cells. Mutations are errors in DNA replication. Substances which cause breaks in DNA strands or otherwise interfere with the orderly sequence of events in DNA replication increase the spontaneous, low rate of errors. The fact that carcinogens are mutagens strongly suggests that cancer is a derangement of DNA functioning in the cell, probably of one or more of its growth-controlling sections. The mutagenesis hypothesis provides the basis for a very useful screening test for potential new carcinogens made by the chemical industry. In this test, devised by Dr. Bruce Ames, liver cells and test bacteria are incorporated into an agar growth medium. The putative carcinogen is applied as a spot and diffuses into the medium. Growth conditions are arranged such that only mutant colonies can grow. The number of colonies and the distance from the spot application at which they can be found are indices of the mutagenic potential of the chemical. The point of the liver cells is to pick up substances that might be converted metabolically into carcinogens. This test does not substitute for animal tests, but it is useful in screening out highly suspicious substances.

The mutagen theory also makes for a plausible role for co-carcinogens, or promoting substances. A mutation can manifest itself only when cells divide, and these irritants are non-specific stimuli for cellular multiplication.

Of course, only a minute minority of all mutant cells will have the particular error that leads to malignancy. In fact, it is probable that in most cases cells do not leap from normalcy to malignancy in one mutational step. Sequential mutations are required, each leading the cell a bit further from normal growth control. Therefore, natural carcinogens act over long periods and repeated exposure is required.

It is currently fashionable to ascribe the bulk of human cancer, perhaps 80 percent, to chemical carcinogenesis, but hard evidence for this figure is lacking. The case for linking smoking and lung cancer is beyond dispute. Strong arguments suggest that the rising incidence of colon cancer in Western countries (as opposed to Africa or Japan) may be due to dietary factors. One particular theory is that diets low in roughage permit a prolonged sojourn of food residues in the colon and favor the growth of organisms capable of converting bile salts into nitrosamines, strongly carcinogenic substances. The high incidence of stomach cancer in the Japanese is speculatively ascribed to high intake of smoked fish, which contains tars. In all of these situations, the essentially random nature of the process of mutation ensures that only some people exposed to carcinogens will develop malignancy. Unless the dose is artificially large, as in laboratory experiments, the majority will be spared. This, together with the fact that other considerations such as genetic constitution enter into the complex pattern of cancer causation, has provided much comfort to the apologists for the tobacco industry. It should not be allowed to obscure the central issue: lung cancer is 30 times more common in heavy smokers than in nonsmokers, and represents a modern epidemic that could be readily prevented.

Viral Carcinogenesis

The observation that viruses isolated from cancer tissue can
sometimes induce the same cancer on injection into another
animal is as old as this century, and has engendered a monu-
mental amount of work on viral carcinogenesis, chiefly in mice.
There is no doubt whatever that viruses can cause cancer. The
question is, how often are they responsible for the "spontaneous" cancers of man? So far there is only a single malignancy in man, the rather rare tumor of the jaw found in African
children and young people, known as Burkitt's lymphoma, where
authorities agree that a virus is an obligatory factor in causation.
Of course, the proponents of tumor virology argue quite plaus-
ibly that the crucial experiment, isolating the virus from the
tumor and injecting it into a susceptible host, cannot be done
in man, and this final proof of viral causation is impossible to
achieve. What can be provided is guilt by association—finding
virus particles or traces of viral genes in a high percentage of
cancers of a particular type. This search, except for Burkitt's
lymphoma, has been rather frustrating in man. Nevertheless,
the various laboratory models that have been built up over the
years are so powerful and so convincing that it would be wise
to keep a very open mind on the matter of human cancer
viruses.

In the laboratory animal, tumor or oncogenic viruses fall
into two broad types. The DNA viruses can infiltrate themselves directly into the genetic material of the host cell. The
RNA tumor viruses contain an enzyme, reverse transcriptase,
which can cause a DNA copy to be made of an RNA blueprint,
thus reversing the normal genetic dogma. In this way, viral
RNA-coded genes can find their way into the cell's nucleus.
Tumor viruses do not, unlike many normal viruses, destroy the
cell which they infect. They need not even continue to multiply

in the host cell. Rather, they become part of the cell's genetic machinery and transform its healthy functioning. Again, we see altered gene functioning as the final common pathway underlying carcinogenesis.

Cancer viruses may be incredibly widespread in the species carrying them and by no means always result in cancer induction. For example, in Burkitt's lymphoma, all patients show the presence of the so-called Epstein-Barr virus genes in the tumor cells. However, this virus is much better known as the cause of the common infection glandular fever or infectious mononucleosis. In fact, half of the adults in most communities have had an infection with Epstein-Barr virus, mostly quite unsymptomatic (subclinical glandular fever). Yet Burkitt's lymphoma is very rare. The probable explanation is that the virus causes cancer only in people of the right genetic constitution, and in the presence of some second causative or promoting factor. There has been speculation that chronic malaria may be the second factor for Burkitt's lymphoma.

Laboratory mice follow another common pattern. For example, the virus responsible for lymphatic leukemia may be ubiquitous in a colony; it is transmitted from parent to offspring via the egg, a process termed vertical transmission. It proliferates widely in the body, without initially harming the cells. Eventually, however, malignancy supervenes, perhaps at one year of age. If viruses are artificially recovered from such leukemic cells and injected into newborn suckling mice of the same strain, these in turn might come down with cancer earlier, say at six months. If this procedure is repeated a sufficient number of times, an extremely powerfully carcinogenic virus strain may eventually be selected. Thus the Friend leukemia virus can cause fatal leukemia three weeks after injection. While such model strains may be a long distance from spontaneous events in nature, they are nevertheless very useful in elucidating the molecular steps by which a virus may gain control over a cell's growth processes. We can learn even more about viruses by observing them in tissue culture. Here, their effects in normal cells manifest themselves quickly and can be studied in great biochemical detail. If it is necessary to prove that virally transformed cells are truly malignant, the infected tissue culture can be injected into an animal host to see if it grows into a tumor. Among the human tumors for which a viral cause is being most avidly sought (on the basis of comparable animal models) are the leukemias and lymphomas, breast cancer and cancer of the uterine cervix. Whatever turns out to be the real role of cancer viruses in humans, it must be remembered that cancer is in no sense an infectious disease. Most likely, the cancer virus will be caught *not* from a cancer sufferer but rather through vertical transmission via egg or milk; or (as in the case of the Epstein-Barr virus) from a person suffering from a mild disease. Even in the laboratory, cancer is not "caught" by one animal from a tumor-bearer, but rather is transmitted in an artificial fashion.

One is frequently asked about the prospects for a cancer vaccine. Unfortunately, the answer must be that this is a long way off. Even when proof is finally obtained that this or that cancer is due to a virus, much debate will ensue as to whether a vaccine against that virus will be safe, effective, and worthwhile. We know the best viral vaccines are live attenuated ones, but how could one ensure that laboratory attenuation also removed oncogenicity? How much money would the public be prepared to spend to vaccinate *all* people so that one in 5000 of them does not develop the particular cancer? These are deep questions which will take ages to answer, particularly given the long latent period of most human cancers.

Radiation-Induced Malignancies

One good way of increasing mutation rates is to expose cells to ionizing radiation such as X-rays or radioactive fallout. Such radiation causes damage to DNA. If very severe, the cell is permanently prevented from dividing; when it attempts to divide it simply commits suicide. If the damage is less severe, the cell can use its enzyme system to repair DNA damage, but the risk of mutations creeping in is considerable. Little wonder, then, that radiation, a powerful mutagen, is also a carcinogen. A tragic example of this was the high incidence of leukemia and other tumors in the early radiologists, who used X-rays and radium without knowing about the side effects.

Even ultraviolet radiation, such as from sunlight, can be mutagenic in sufficient doses. It is generally believed that the high incidence of skin cancers in white Australians reflects the effects of excess ultraviolet rays on skins not sufficiently protected by melanin pigment.

There has been a great deal of argument about whether the amount of damage to DNA, and thus the chance of cancer or of damaging the germ cells and causing congenital abnormalities in the offspring, is directly proportional to radiation dose over the whole range from "background" radiation to lethal levels; or whether there is some threshold for damage, below which level the cell can perform effective DNA repair. If the former is true, then *any* level of radiation, such as dental X-rays or even trace amounts of fallout from nuclear testing, increases the mutational burden at community level. If the latter is the case, our concern about minimal radiation levels is unjustified. The experimental evidence peters out below about one-fiftieth of a lethal dose—a level still associated with some slight mutagenesis—but the radiation loads of practical concern are fiftyfold lower again. French scientists defending their government's decision to continue atmospheric nuclear testing in the Pacific during the early 1970s were vocal in their descriptions of elaborate and specialized DNA repair mechanisms in cells and argued for a threshold, but even they had to agree that the point had not been scientifically proven. Eventually, aroused public opinion forced France to perform its testing explosions underground. As far as medical X-ray or isotope scanning procedures are concerned, no pains are spared today in minimizing radiation dose, and the possible theoretical risks are negligible in relation to the potential benefits.

Other Biological Factors in Carcinogenesis

Growth is a complex process and can be deranged in a wide variety of ways. Thus, while we have discussed the most flagrant carcinogenic influences, others are known and still others will certainly be discovered in the future. One vitally important factor is hormone levels. Hormones are the body's messengers bringing signals for growth or metabolic activity from an endocrine gland to a target tissue. The growth of many cells is hormone-dependent. For example, at puberty when a surge of sex hormones is released, they trigger growth in sex organs and other tissues such as the beard, pubic hair, and the breast. Some cancers, particularly at relatively early stages, are not yet capable of entirely independent growth. They too are hormone-dependent. In the case of metastatic breast cancer, a dramatic response may be obtained by removing the ovaries and adrenals, thereby drastically lowering levels of sex steroids. Alternatively, benefit may follow the administration of testosterone, the male sex hormone with an opposite influence. Prostate cancer in men can often be effectively manipulated hormonally. Useful as these treatments are, eventually most cancers break through and reach a stage of hormone independence. Disastrous effects can follow if tissues are exposed to hormones before they should be. For example, when I was a medical student 25 years ago, it was quite common to treat threatened abortion with high levels of estrogens (female sex hormones). It is hard to know how effective this was in maintaining the pregnancy, but it certainly exposed the fetus to abnormally high levels of estrogens, which readily cross the placenta. A distressing number of female children born after such treatment turn up in their teens with cancer of the vagina—a rare tumor at any age and previously unknown in teenagers. Clearly the growth stimulus at an inappropriate time had sown the seeds of carcinogenicity.

There are numerous other examples of excessive stimuli to growth ending up as cancer. For instance, ulcerative colitis is an inflammatory disease in which ulcers appear in the mucous lining of the gut and constantly need to be repaired. Colon cancer is a well-known and not infrequent complication of ulcerative colitis. Skin cancers can develop in the edges of varicose or diabetic ulcers, where cells are continuously striving to repair the skin defect. Still, these and similar examples are not entirely straightforward, as constant *normal* stimulation of cell growth will not cause cancer; the gardener, no matter how he toils, will not get cancer in his calluses, or the long-distance runner in the muscles of his heart. We have a great deal yet to learn about normal control processes in cellular growth and their aberrations.

Tumor-Specific Antigens and Immune Surveillance

The cancer cell differs chemically from normal cells, and frequently this difference can be recognized by the immune system of the host. In particular, most experimentally induced tumors display one or more molecules on their surface which are anti-genic. These are referred to as tumor-specific or tumor-associated antigens. When these antigens evoke a brisk killer T cell response, as they frequently do, they are referred to as tumor-associated transplantation antigens, or TATA. Cells rendered cancerous by oncogenic viruses display a variety of virus-specific TATA on their surface, some of which actually represent portions of the virus particle budding off the cell membrane, but others of which, though virally coded, exist as cell surface constituents even in cells not actively producing virus. As these TATA are coded for by viral nucleic acids, all cells infected by the same virus will display the same spectrum of TATA.

Such is not the case for many carcinogen-induced malignancies. As these appear to be the result of mutations, and as mutation is a very random affair, different cancers will display different TATA. This is schematically summarized in Figures 20–1 and 20–2. Yet, as well as these *individual-specific* TATA, many carcinogen-induced malignancies also carry antigens common to all tumors of that particular histological type.

A third important group of TATA are the so-called oncofetal antigens. It turns out that many tumors share antigens with normal tissue of embryos. This has been taken as a strong point in favor of the old theory that cancer really represents a reversion to an embryonic pattern of cell behavior. The oncofetal antigens are widely cross-reactive; for example in the mouse, plasma cell tumors and fibrosarcomas may both share antigens with fetal liver cells.

If tumors are antigenic, why do they ever grow? Why are they not rejected by the immune system before they reach clinical size? One answer is provided by the proponents of the *immune surveillance* hypothesis. This states that one of the prime jobs which evolution has given to the immune system, particularly the T cell system, is to seek out and destroy "altered self," or cells which are somewhat different from normal cells. These would include cells that have undergone malignant trans-

CANCER VIRUS ACTS (e.g. Leukaemia)

Transformed Cell Grows
Selectively

All Tumors Caused by Same Virus Are Antigenically Similar

Figure 20–1. Common tumor-specific antigens in two tumors caused by the same virus.

 CARCINOGEN ACTS (e.g. Cigarette Smoke)

Mutant Cells Grows Selectively

All Tumors Caused by Same Carcinogen Are Antigenically Different

Figure 20–2. Different tumor-specific antigens in two tumors caused by the same chemical carcinogen.

formation. Clinical cancer results only when immune surveillance fails. It represents the tip of an iceberg, and the whole cancer problem would be much worse if there were no immune system. Most workers agree that the immune surveillance hypothesis has merit for virus-induced malignancies, which are increased in incidence and appear earlier in immunosuppressed animals. It is more dubious in the case of carcinogen-induced malignancies, where increases after immunosuppression are not seen. However, it is noted that tumors which arise early after a high dose of carcinogen are often strongly antigenic, perhaps because the carcinogen suppresses immune surveillance. Tumors that arise late after a repeated low-dose administration of carcinogen (a situation more akin to the human one) usually have weak TATA. Spontaneous tumors, which arise in mice not intentionally treated with any carcinogen, have the lowest immunogenicity of all. This is interpreted as a bad sign for the would-be tumor immunotherapist, but is consistent with the notion of immune surveillance "polishing off" the antigenic tumors.

Some workers believe that the immune surveillance notion has been "oversold." They explain the emergence of an antigenic tumor in the following way. The initial transforming event occurs in only one cell, and the few TATA molecules which it sheds off are clearly too few numerically to signal the immune system effectively. As the tumor grows, more antigen is released, but the immune response will always be quantitative, not infinite. It is therefore a "race" between the inherent growth drive of the tumor and the aggressivity of the immune attack. There are no a priori reasons why the lymphocytes should win the race. In fact, the tumor has many mechanisms available to it to elude immune defenses, such as inaccessibility of cells to invading lymphocytes, emergence of immunoresistant cell lines lacking TATA or not readily susceptible to cytotoxic attack, and "blindfolding" of killer cells by shed TATA jamming into lymphocyte receptors before the cell gets to the tumor. The situation with respect to a growing cancer is quite different from that pertaining when the investigator injects tumor cells into an animal *pre-immunized* against that tumor. Here, the cards are stacked in the host's favor and the preexistent immune state may frequently eliminate the grafted tumor cells.

Tumor-Destructive Mechanisms in Immunized Recipients

An animal which has been immunized against a particular tumor and its set of TATA has several mechanisms available to it which are capable of hastening the destruction of dividing tumor cells later injected into the same animal. Frequently it is difficult to sort out which one is of the greatest importance *in vivo*. Antibody molecules against TATA may cause tumor cell lysis by complement fixation. Antibodies may also coat tumor cells and make them palatable to macrophages. Cytotoxic killer T cells against TATA have been noted in many tumors, and are probably of great importance in limiting tumor spread. A curious mechanism is one involving both antibodies and a lymphoid cell known as a K cell. This cell, which is neither a B cell nor a T cell, can bind antibodies firmly to its surface via an Fc receptor. If anti-TATA is present, this attached antibody will "steer" the K cell into contact with tumor cells, and, even though the K cell itself has no specificity for the TATA in question, killing ensues. The K cell has acquired its specificity vicariously by grabbing hold of specific antibody. Recently, in normal, unimmunized animals a population of "spontaneous" killer cells have been identified which have the capacity to kill a wide variety of cells in the absence of antibodies. Also, it is known that macrophages which have been activated by factors derived from antigenically stimulated T cells can exert a nonspecific killer action on tumors. The future alone will tell which of these many mechanisms correlate with true protection, and which are of more theoretical interest.

One of the disappointing features of clinical tumor immunology has been that our knowledge of human TATA has not advanced nearly as quickly as that of TATA in animal models. Claims for the discovery of TATA in human cancers such as leukemias, malignant melanomas, and sarcomas are frequent but confirmations have been slow in coming forward. An unequivocal cell membrane antigen has been identified in human lymphoblastic leukemia, and some authors believe the evidence is becoming solid for melanoma. Many cancers secrete an antigen known as CEA (carcino-embryonic antigen), but as this does not evoke an immune attack and can, in fact, be present in quite large amounts in certain diseases other than cancer, it is not really a TATA. The failure yet to find convincing TATA for common cancers such as those of the lung, breast, colon, and uterus is galling. It may mirror, in part, the experimental observation that "spontaneous" tumors in experimental animals are of low immunogenicity.

Treatment of Cancer

The three conventional linchpins of cancer treatment are surgery, radiotherapy, and chemotherapy. Surgery is frequently curative, even for serious malignancies such as those of the colon or breast. In these tumors, if the operation is performed before any spread to local lymph nodes can be noted, the cure rate in the best series approaches 80 percent. This is not to say that not a single malignant cell has escaped from the confines of the primary tumor and has reached a lymph node or the bloodstream. Once the primary tumor is removed, these microscopic deposits may well be dealt with by immune mechanisms or other growth-controlling influences in the host. Even cancer cells are not 100 percent efficient in establishing themselves in a foreign environment! Obviously, the results of cancer surgery will be influenced by early diagnosis (which in turn depends on when the tumor causes symptoms or visible signs), and even more by the natural history of the tumor. If it is one in which metastatic spread occurs very early, surgery by itself will hold out little hope.

Radiotherapy, or the use of large doses of X-rays or other forms of ionizing radiation to kill dividing cells, is the primary treatment of choice in some cancers. For example, it is very effective for the lowly malignant tumor basal cell carcinoma of the skin. It may also be preferred for tumors inaccessible to the surgeon's knife. However, the primary cure of cancer represents only a small part of the role of radiotherapy. It finds its widest use for pain relief and palliation (though not cure) in advanced metastatic cancer.

Chemotherapy is the use of drugs which act on cancer cells, usually through inhibiting cell division by one means or another. Cancer cells, on the average, divide more frequently than normal cells and are hit more heavily by mitotic poisons. Of course, these drugs are dangerous and can also damage bone marrow, lymphoid cells, and others. Therefore, dosage has to be very carefully controlled. Not long ago, cancer chemotherapy was thought of mainly in terms of palliation for late cancer. Gradually, however, this picture is changing and physicians are actually achieving long-term remissions with drugs. The first field to benefit from the more aggressive approach to chemotherapy was acute lymphoblastic leukemia, the common form of childhood leukemia. It is now standard to use several drugs in combination in attempts to destroy the last leukemic cell. The chances are that if a particular cell is a mutant resistant to drug A, it will remain susceptible to drug B, so combination chemotherapy has a better chance of coping with mutants than a single drug. Also, the eight or ten commonly used drugs differ in their mode of action, some even being capable of harming cancer cells that are not in mitotic cycle. Now that experience has built up concerning combination chemotherapy, we are at last daring to speak about cures of acute leukemia. Certainly, some children have been entirely symptom-free for 10 years.

More recently, vigorous chemotherapy of solid tumors (as opposed to the widely dispersed leukemias and lymphomas) has given promising results. For example, in Stage 2 breast cancer, where metastases have already reached the local lymph node, the prognosis for patients treated with surgery and radiation is bad, and one half are either dead or suffering from widespread metastases after three years. For patients treated with surgery and combination chemotherapy, some 85 percent are entirely free of symptoms after three years. It is too early to tell whether this means real cure, but the encouraging results are creating a climate where more doctors are turning to chemotherapy at early, rather than late, stages of tumor progression.

Immunotherapy of Tumors

Treatment of cancer by attempts to strengthen the immune attack against the cancer cell represents a recent development in clinical oncology, with a history of only about 10 years. It is too early to assess its final place in cancer management. Most of the large, well-controlled clinical trials that have been published so far have given, at best, marginally better results for the group given immunotherapy plus conventional treatment than the group given conventional treatment alone. Still, many clinicians, on the basis of their individual experience, believe strongly in immunotherapy, particularly for leukemia and malignant melanoma. Also, one keeps hearing of as yet unpublished clinical trials "in the pipeline" that show more clear-cut benefits. Therefore it is still possible to maintain a cautious optimism about immunotherapy.

There are two main themes underlying the many different protocols employed in cancer immunotherapy. The first is an attempt at vaccination with cancer antigens as such. Tumor cells from the patient or from a patient with a similar malignancy are irradiated, so that they cannot divide any more, and sometimes treated with enzymes designed to "expose" TATA more completely on the cell surface. Then the tumor cells are injected and the patient is simultaneously given an adjuvant to heighten immune responsiveness. The two most commonly used adjuvants are BCG vaccine (or fractions of BCG bacteria) and killed *Corynebacterium parvum* preparations. The hope of this specific tumor immunotherapy is to raise killer T cells and cytotoxic antibodies against tumor cells. The second approach is to rely on immune adjuvants alone, in the hope both that residual tumor cells within the patient will provide the antigen source, and that a *nonspecific* rise in immune activity may help to destroy cancer cells, perhaps by creating angry macrophages.

One interesting variant of immune therapy has been applied to the problem of multiple and extensive skin cancers, apparently with frequent success. The patient is first sensitized to some immunogenic chemical, such as dinitrochlorobenzene, and develops delayed hypersensitivity to it. Then the chemical is painted on the skin lesion, which rapidly becomes inflamed and angry. Apparently, tumor cells are extensively killed during this phase, as, when the inflammation subsides after four weeks or so, the tumor has disappeared. Curiously, inflammatory changes and tumor destruction can occur even over some cancers *not* painted with the chemical. The mechanism for this phenomenon, in which cancer cells are killed as "innocent bystanders" during an irrelevant immune response to a test antigen, is not fully understood. Perhaps the violent T cell response to the chemical arms macrophages to kill tumor cells.

Perhaps the inflammation causes a pulse of tumor antigens to be released with a sudden surge in antitumor killer T cell levels and resultant tumor destruction. This mechanism could explain how unpainted areas containing tumor cells (and thus targets for the wandering killer cells' action) could also benefit. The same general approach has been used to treat skin metastases of tumors from other organs such as the breast, but here the success rate is much lower.

Adjuvants currently in use are somewhat toxic and not well understood. There would be advantages in finding a defined, simple chemical which could specifically heighten immune responsiveness. There have been claims that a drug initially used to kill parasitic worms has immunopotentiating action. This drug, levamisole, is under trial in a variety of clinical situations but it has generally been disappointing. A number of other compounds, such as a nucleic acid analogue called poly-AU and a fraction of bacterial wall called lipid A, demonstrate strong adjuvant action in experimental animals, but have not yet been used in man.

Whatever definitive role finally emerges for human tumor immunotherapy, the following guiding principle will certainly hold true. The body's immune attack will always be a strictly quantitative affair—so many lymphocytes battling against so many cancer cells. Therefore, immunotherapy will stand its best chance if used when the tumor load is low, for example, immediately after surgery or chemotherapy. It is too much to expect the immune system to cope with huge, well-established tumor masses by itself. From this point of view, immunotherapy must be viewed not as an isolated treatment but rather as an adjunct to more conventional therapy. If it does turn out to be powerful in ridding the body of tiny microscopic rests of cancer cells not visible to the surgeon, this alone would more than justify the high research investment being made at present.

Immunology in Cancer Diagnosis

If further research reveals more human TATA, immunology should be of great use in early cancer diagnosis and classification. For example, antibodies to the various TATA could be rendered fluorescent or radioactive, and biopsies of suspicious lumps could be examined to see if they took up the antibodies specifically, i.e., possessed the TATA concerned. Best of all would be a blood test for cancer, capable of picking up the minuscule amounts of TATA which might be shed off the surface of a small tumor and reach the bloodstream.

There are currently two proteins produced by cancers for which blood tests already exist. The first is CEA, or carcino-embryonic antigen, which, as we have mentioned, is not strictly a TATA. Though tests can now pick up 0.005 micrograms of CEA per milliliter of serum, the levels in *very early* cancer are still lower than this. Furthermore, patients suffering from other diseases may show raised CEA levels, and thus the test has not lived up to its early promise as a screening test for cancer. Nevertheless, it is useful in patient management. If a cancer patient has raised CEA levels, and these do not fall rapidly after surgery, this means that not all the tumor has been removed, and can even convince the surgeon to go and have a "second look." If CEA does disappear, but reappears some months later, this is a strong indication that metastases have grown up somewhere.

The second protein is also one made normally in fetal life. It is called AFP, or alpha-fetoprotein, and it can be indicative of the presence of liver cancer. It is hoped that these two tests are only early harbingers of many more to come as our knowledge of human tumor immunology increases.

Whether the immune system turns out to be of great practical importance in human cancer or not, it is sure that major con-

tinuing effort in the cancer field will go into the question of prevention. In particular, as the case for individual carcinogens
gets stronger, the pressures for their removal from the human
environment will grow. Surely society's first major effort should
be in the field of smoking. About one in ten of all heavy
smokers will die of lung cancer, and two in ten from some other
disease aggravated by smoking. The heavy smoker shortens his
or her life by five to twelve years. Is it any wonder that so
many doctors have given up cigarettes over the last decade?
Sweden has made a conscious political decision to create a
smokeless society by the year 2000. Other countries should
follow this lead.

21

TROPICAL DISEASES

WHILE infectious diseases have been largely conquered in the developed countries, many millions of people, especially those living in tropical regions, suffer and die from communicable diseases. Not only do bacterial and viral diseases take a heavy toll, but an added burden is provided by parasitic diseases, caused by single-celled organisms or lowly worms which invade the tissues and persist for months or years. While literally dozens of kinds of parasites afflict humans, each having its own particular life cycle and spectrum of pathological effects on the host, a common feature in most cases is that transmission is mediated by some vector, be this a mosquito, a fly, a bug, or a snail. One reason for parasitic disease being so much more common in the tropics is that climatic conditions favor the breeding of these vectors. Another, of course, is that many of the affected countries have been cut off from the mainstream of world social and economic progress. A kind of vicious cycle of poverty, hunger, disease, and low economic performance conspires to keep public health and sanitation at a low level. However, though existing knowledge and technology could materially lessen the burden of parasitism if fully coordinated and exploited, the technical tools now available to control certain of the diseases are inadequate and new tools will have to be devised through research. In particular, no vaccine yet exists against any human parasitic disease.

Parasitic diseases can lead to early death, but more often they cause chronic, long-lasting illnesses that sap vitality and lower work efficiency. Therefore, apart from the human distress they cause, the tropical diseases represent a major obstacle to economic development and social progress.

Some Key Villains of Tropical Pathology

Three examples will serve to illustrate the type of problem which parasitic diseases represent. Among the worst villains are malaria, schistosomiasis, and filariasis.

Malaria is still one of the most widespread diseases in the world. It affects at least a quarter of a billion people, and it is estimated that just in Africa south of the Sahara, one million children die of it each year. Malaria, like many parasitic infections, is not really a single disease but occurs in four different forms according to the particular species of Plasmodium parasite involved. Plasmodia are a type of protozoon or single-celled organism. After initial injection into man via the bite of an infected mosquito, they undergo quite a complex life cycle. At first, the cell injected by the mosquito bite (the sporozoite), goes underground in the liver. Then it emerges as a merozoite and parasitizes the red cells. Within the red cells, extensive multiplication of merozoites takes place, and progeny are released when a red cell bursts which can then enter and destroy further red cells. When an acute attack is finally overcome, the parasites may once again flee to the liver, only to re-emerge at some future time. Of course, in an endemic area, re-infection via mosquito bites can occur at any time and re-initiate the cycle. However, eventually a partial immunity does supervene.

The main burden of the attack falls on the red cells, and acute malaria is accompanied by extensive red cell destruction, fever, and anemia. In the more chronic phase, enlargement of the spleen, which has to do all the work of clearing the burst red cells from the blood stream, is a constant feature. Also, the concomitant occurrence of antigen and antibodies within the body leads to immune complex formation, as a result of which kidneys and many other organs can be damaged. The most malignant form of malaria, caused by *Plasmodium falciparum*, is frequently fatal.

In some countries, malaria has been eliminated through control of mosquitoes alone. This was achieved essentially by eliminating the particular species of mosquitoes capable of carrying malaria through the use of insecticides, chiefly DDT. In other countries, the opportunities for mosquito breeding are so extensive that it can be forcefully stated that insecticides alone will never fully cope with the problem.

Two serious public health dilemmas in malaria are the increasing incidences of parasite resistance to chloroquine, the best prophylactic drug, and of mosquito resistance to DDT.

Schistosomiasis

Schistosomiasis, also known as bilharziasis or snail fever, is a chronic debilitating group of diseases caused by small worms known as trematodes or flukes. Four species of *Schistosoma* commonly infect man, and damage particular target organs. The most widespread is *Schistosoma mansoni*, which affects chiefly the bowel and abdomen. Other species damage the urinary tract or the liver. The life cycle of schistosomes involves the release of parasite eggs by infected people, via the urine or feces, into fresh water such as ponds or lakes. Here, the eggs hatch into larvae which infect freshwater snails. These, in turn, favor multiplication and release large numbers of free-swimming forms called cercariae. These penetrate the skin of people wading in the infested water and work their way into small blood vessels. Maturation into adult worms of both sexes takes place, and, in a very cozy domestic arrangement, adult pairs of worms can lie side by side in the blood vessel for years. Much of the damage in schistosomiasis is done by the eggs which are laid in huge numbers over this period. Some are excreted, but many lodge in the tissues where they excite a chronic inflammation and finally scarring, fibrosis, and even cancer.

Artificial lakes and irrigation canals are prime breeding grounds for the schistosome, and the disease has increased considerably in Egypt since the building of the Aswan dam. By a quixotic turn of fate, major development programs have caused as great a problem as they have solved!

Molluscicides are an important weapon in the fight against schistosomiasis, as is collection and killing of snails under some circumstances, as in China. Schistosomes themselves can be killed within the human host by certain anti-helminthic drugs, but most of those currently available are toxic and not really suitable for mass administration. Clean, uncontaminated water supplies provide a clear-cut answer if accompanied by avoidance of old habits, but it will be decades until these are universally available in many countries.

Elephantiasis and River Blindness

Filariasis is a group of diseases caused by filarial worms that live in lymphatic vessels. They obstruct lymph flow, and can cause the hideous buildup of fluid and eventually chronic swelling of limbs or genitals known as elephantiasis. One particularly vicious form of filariasis is called onchocerciasis or river blindness. The adult worms breed embryos known as microfilariae, which can invade the eyes in their teeming millions. This causes progressive deterioration of vision and eventually blindness. The vector of onchocerciasis is a species of blackfly, which injects onchocerca larvae into man and initiates this merciless disease. It is most appropriately named *Simulium damnosum*. It breeds only in fast-flowing, oxygen-rich water, that is, in the very regions which are most suitable for agriculture. Insecticides can destroy blackfly larvae in their breeding grounds and a major onchocerciasis control program based on insecticide spraying has been launched in seven African countries in the Volta River basin. This approach can do nothing for the sufferer from established disease.

Drugs do exist which kill the microfilariae of onchocerca resident in the patient's eyes. However, effective treatment can cause an acute and severe flare-up of ocular damage. The probable reason is that as the microfilariae are killed, there is a substantial, pulsatile release of antigens, and antibodies plus T lymphocytes flock to the area and cause inflammatory damage. This can be controlled through cortisone drops, at least to a degree. We need better drugs in filariasis, however, and these will form an important part of the control program in Africa. As the patients themselves represent a reservoir of infection until freed of disease, it is estimated that insecticiding might have to continue for 20 years to control vectors until the patient parasite pool falls to an insignificant level. It is hard to believe that such a long program will not encounter major problems of vector resistance or ecological complications. Suitable mass drug administration could shorten the requisite period by decreasing the human reservoir of parasites.

Other parasitic diseases of great importance include trypanosomiasis, which in its African form causes sleeping sickness and in its South American form the heart-damaging Chagas' disease; leishmaniasis, which causes tropical sores and also fatal visceral infections; hookworm, which infects the small bowel and causes anemia; and amebic infections that can cause dysentery or liver abscesses. As well as these, bacterial infections such as leprosy, cholera, and typhoid and virus diseases such as yellow fever and many enteric infections, continue to take a devastating toll.

Immunity in Parasitic Disease

In many parasitic infections, repeated re-exposure to the same causal agent is the norm. The question is why does not the immune system learn to cope with both the initial parasites and these re-invasions? The chief reason is that over millions of years of evolution, parasites have learnt a variety of tricks to foil the immune systems of their hosts. In fact, it can be argued that the most successful parasites are those that evoke a partial immune response. If the host's immune response were too good, the parasite might soon die out for lack of susceptible hosts. If immune defense were totally absent, the parasites might kill the host and soon run out of victims, and therefore perish.

Indeed, partial immunity is frequently observed in parasitism, though it must be admitted that our knowledge of immune mechanisms in these diseases is far less detailed than it ought to be. The person who has lived for 15 years in an area of high malarial endemicity and without benefit of drug prophylaxis will certainly react differently to his next bite by an infected mosquito than a person exposed for the first time. Similarly, re-infestation by schistosomes is said to cause a lesser degree of egg production per entering cercaria than in a naive host. However, in most parasitic diseases, immunity does not sterilize; it fails to get rid of the parasite altogether.

Parasites perform a variety of tricks. They may coat them-selves or their eggs with a layer of host material, and thus shield themselves from immune attack. They may undergo antigenic variation, a fascinating phenomenon whereby the parasite changes its antigenic coat to a new form. They may pursue a major part of their life cycles sequestered inside cells and inaccessible to antibodies or killer T cells. They may exhibit a tough skin that easily repels the puny lymphocytes' charge. They may shelter themselves behind a thick-walled cyst. All of these and many more behavioral twists are designed to frustrate host resistance.

In the face of these mechanisms, is it realistic to think of antiparasite vaccines? The answer is indubitably yes, as the feasibility of some vaccines has already been established in veterinary medicine. The point is that in the overall life cycle, there should be some Achilles' heel, some phase more readily amenable to immune destruction than the total parasite burden. For example, in malaria, two susceptibility points might be: a) just after entry of the sporozoite from the mosquito and before its disappearance into the liver; b) the brief period between the rupture of a red cell and the release of merozoites and their entry into the next red cell. While the problem will vary from disease to disease, it should not be impossible to define antigens crucially important for some of these steps, and to build a vaccine up around well understood principles. Just as in cancer, the immunological approach may well not succeed in established cases with a large parasite burden. Rather, the vaccine should be designed to prevent the establishment of the initial infection. Only then will the cards be stacked firmly in the host's favor.

Major Obstacles for the Vaccine Approach to Parasitism

No one believes that the development of any antiparasite vaccine will be an easy task. First of all, vaccines require a reliable source of large quantities of antigen in reasonably pure form. As parasites do not grow on artificial growth media, tissue culture approaches, frequently of a highly specialized and sophisticated nature, will have to be developed. In April, 1976, Dr. William Trager of the Rockefeller University in New York announced his success in culturing *Plasmodium falciparum* continuously for three months in human red blood cells—a major triumph. Similar encouraging results have recently been achieved for trypanosomiasis.

Second, parasites are much more complex biochemically than viruses and bacteria, and contain many more antigens. The host mounts an immune attack against a myriad of parasite molecules, but only a few of the many antibodies produced may be helpful in protection. For example, antibodies against the skin of a two-foot-long worm may be quite useless, whereas antibodies against some vital receptor molecule important in the penetration of the larval form of the same worm through a vessel wall may be of critical importance. Clearly there is a major job ahead in the progressive definition, analysis, and purification of parasite antigens.

Third, antigenic variation presents a challenge. It may be possible to define common, core antigens not susceptible to variation, which may be less exposed on the parasite cell's surface, yet sufficiently crucial to make a susceptible target.

As with all vaccines, antigen dosage will be a problem in parasite vaccines. Compared with microbes, the bulk of parasite cells is large, and the injection of whole killed organisms or of irradiated parasites which cannot multiply or give offspring, represents a great load of foreign proteins on the host. This involves the possibility of nasty vaccine reactions, perhaps acceptable in veterinary medicine but not in humans. We have already noted that we do not require antibody formation against irrelevant material inside the parasite cells, and antigen purification steps seem almost inevitable if enough of the *right* antigen is to go into the vaccine. On the other hand, in some cases, live, attenuated vaccines may represent a better approach. Then the huge problem of effectiveness of the attenuation step will have to be overcome, as it has been for many viral vaccines.

The above may sound somewhat tentative and even speculative. This is because of the inordinate number of unknowns not yet revealed by research. There is a great requirement to explore in depth various laboratory models of the human parasitic diseases. Scientists are now developing these, using both the smaller laboratory rodents and various subhuman primates. Also, far more clinical research needs to be done on the patients' responses to parasites; on the correlations of various antibodies or T cell activities with protection; on the influence of immune response genes on disease susceptibility; on the number of undesirable, immunopathological results of immune reactions to parasite invasion. Underlying all of this, there will have to be a growing body of basic knowledge of immunological features of parasites and hosts provided by fundamental immunology research.

Future Challenges for Other Approaches to Parasitism

It would be foolish to rely on immunology alone to solve the problems of parasitism. Chemotherapy has a huge role to play, both with respect to prophylactics suitable for mass administration and in treatment of actual infections. The search for new, better, cheaper, safer, and more effective drugs should be accelerated. Control of vectors will remain important, and research should come up with ecological methods of vector eradication as alternatives to pesticides. For example, fish capable of eating mosquito larvae are already in experimental use. Environmental measures will be of major significance in particular localities. Epidemiology has much to contribute towards increasing our knowledge of prevalence rates, and of ecological and genetic factors influencing disease severity. Improving overall nutrition will be helpful in increasing individual resistance to parasites. Operational research will be important in optimizing the use of existing tools. Cost-benefit considerations are of paramount importance for any health measure in developing countries, and will also be a necessary prelude to the introduction of new tools provided by more basic research. Finally, any general improvement in standards of living, levels of health education, and patterns of primary health care delivery cannot help but improve the outlook in parasitism.

The World Health Organization has recently launched a special program for research and training in tropical diseases. The aim is the eventual conquest of the five most important groups of parasitic diseases plus leprosy; and the building up of an improved research capacity in the Third World through training and institution-strengthening activities, having their initial focus in Africa. This program has been identified as one of six priority areas in the Organization's work over the next decade. It is conceived as a giant step towards rectifying what has been a clear example of disordered global priorities. The new biology, with its fantastic advances in understanding of cell and molecular functioning, is being widely applied in research aimed at the conquest of diseases of importance to the rich countries. In contrast, the research effort in tropical diseases has, in recent years, been poorly funded and poorly coordinated, with evidence of a slackening rather than an intensification of effort. The WHO program will tap formidable human resources in both the developed and developing world; it will include not only parasitologists but leading fundamental scientists from various disciplines. They will plan and coordinate the research, and a network of collaborating laboratories will ensure its performance. This wonderful example of international cooperation is deserving of widespread interest and support.

22

CONCLUSIONS

MOST of our discussions in this book have related to research achievements in immunology over the last 20 years. While this kind of approach has the advantage of bringing one close to the cutting edge of knowledge in the field, it also has some drawbacks. Chief among these is the fact of exposure to so many areas where information is incomplete and even conceptual analysis vague and unsatisfactory. There are many areas where answers to the most fundamental problems still elude us. What is the biochemical basis of T cell–B cell interaction? Why do some people develop allergies? What is the basic cause of autoimmune disease? What is the real purpose of the major histocompatibility complex? Is tumor immunology an area of real promise?

If you have read the book with interest, some of these questions will be gnawing at you still. The reasons are not hard to find: these are the unsolved issues engaging the skills of research scientists the world over. They will be solved, one by one, but as they are, the new insights gained will spawn new questions that clamor just as urgently to be answered, for this is the way of science. Part of the riddle of man's unending quest

for knowledge of himself and of the world around him is em-
bodied in this spiral relationship. Research leads to knowledge,
and a big component of this new knowledge is to allow the
delineation and description of a new area of ignorance. Researchers themselves recognize this truth intuitively; laymen
may find it more difficult to accept. I suspect most laymen
would be surprised at how anxious scientists are to talk to each
other about new problems, new questions raised by recent
research—much more exciting stuff than the already solved
previous problem, which, once accepted and assimilated, quickly
becomes "old hat." From the layman's point of view, the "new
ignorance" is really only a side-reaction of the main process
of the generation of knowledge. The scientist and the layman
are both right. The full relationship is really a cyclical one, as
shown by the following diagram.

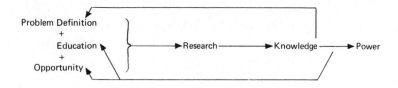

The end-product of the cyclical reaction is power, as every
government in the world has realized. Science and technology
are among the prized new currencies of international politics.
The power generated by scientific research has not always been
put to enlightened use. This is sometimes cited as an argument
against an increased committal of the community's resources to
research. However, any attempt to block the march of scientific
progress by legislative action, no matter how enlightened or
well motivated, is doomed to failure for two reasons. First,
international accords on limitation of research are difficult to
achieve and still harder to enforce. Inspiring though the limitations imposed on biological warfare have been, one wonders
how effectively the negotiations would have proceeded if di-

rected against strategically central areas like nuclear warfare. The best examples of international agreements are those emerging voluntarily from within science itself, such as restrictions on research in recombinant DNA agreed to at the 1975 Asilomar Conference. Second, in the longer term it is against man's nature and the course of history to back away from sources of new knowledge and power. Clearly, governments have a role in stepping in if scientists are not pursuing society's goals. Here, the solution is not to suppress or restrict research, but to channel scientific energies into areas of perceived human benefit. As the bulk of today's research is government-financed, fiscal tactics can achieve this without embarrassment to scientific freedom. To develop enlightened scientific policies, governments will need much help from scientists and will have to understand better the nexus between pure and applied research. Indeed, one of the chief aims of scientific education is to improve society's capacity to comprehend the power and the limits of science. One of the awesome truths about present-day civilization is that man must learn to live with his ability to generate his own instant extinction. This task is not made easier by ostrich-like pleadings for a deceleration in scientific research. Rather, man must look to science and to the new generation of leaders steeped in a knowledge of the world in the scientific era for a solution to the problems generated by his own aggressiveness, curiosity, and greed.

Another criticism leveled specifically at medical science is the contribution which it is making to the problem of large numbers of aged people in society. Certainly the proportion of "over 65s" in the community is greater today than ever before, and part of this is due to medical advances. However, this criticism rapidly collapses when subjected to detailed scrutiny. The main reason for more people surviving to old age is the prevention of death among people who have not yet reached it. Surely even the most Malthusian of observers would not wish to quarrel with this result of scientific progress. Even when we come to medical care of the aged, a much less important contribution to longevity from a statistical point of view, there are indeed few who would be prepared to deny the most advanced and elaborate care to their own dear ones. Once this is acknowledged, it becomes evident that good medical care facilities ought to be available to all aged people. We thus reach the broad conclusion that most of the problems raised by medical and biological science are inevitable side-products, which must be accepted and coped with constructively, but cannot be validly raised as arguments against further work in the area.

In the preceding chapter we looked at some health problems in developing countries. It is often argued that conquest of endemic diseases in these countries will worsen the population explosion and do more harm than good. This also represents spurious reasoning. People will adopt birth control on a wide scale only when they have achieved a sufficient level of education and affluence, and good health is a paramount prerequisite for this. How can one expect an Indian villager to limit his family to two, when he knows that able-bodied sons represent his only security in old age, and that half of his fellow people die as infants or children? Obviously research on better and more varied methods of birth control, ethically and aesthetically acceptable to diverse cultures, is vitally important, but conquest of disease in the Third World must proceed hand in hand with implementation of birth control measures.

It is hoped that there have been two pervading themes throughout the book, which we can now reiterate. The first is that practical medicine and basic biological science are inextricably interwoven. Observation of any typical immunological research establishment in the late 1970s provides many compelling illustrations of this fact. For example, at The Walter and Eliza Hall Institute of Medical Research two out of our five working units have a primary commitment to the understanding, and eventually the cure, of disease processes. These are the Clinical Research Unit and the Cancer Research Unit. The remaining three—Cellular Immunology, Experimental Pathology, Biochemistry, and Biophysics—address themselves mainly to gaining increased understanding of the functioning of the normal immune system. Yet there is daily interchange and cross-stimulation between all the units, and a substantial proportion of the technical papers from the Institute have co-authors from two or more units. Rarely is it possible to draw a line between "pure clinical" and "pure basic" research; most projects have a component of each. Moreover, if we do arbitrarily divide immunology into clinical and theoretical halves, we soon reach the conclusion that many of the key developments in one half have depended utterly on some happening in the other. At the present time, immunology represents perhaps an extreme example of this potential for cross-fertilization between the clinic and the laboratory, physiology being its only rival in this regard. On the other hand, this is a pattern for progress which is becoming an increasingly prominent feature of many of the biosciences.

The second theme has been that of immunology as a moving front which encompasses and forms bridges between many separate disciplines. Biophysics, chemistry, biochemistry, basic cell biology, physiology, genetics, anatomy, embryology, microbiology, pathology, surgery, and medicine have all entered our orbit in one way or another in these pages. There is much talk about a "communications gap" between the various scientific disciplines of our day. Indeed, highly specialized facets of immunology or any other branch of biological science may be of little interest to all nonimmunologists. However, general principles which emerge in a "gap-filling," interdisciplinary subject like immunology can have great value in achieving a wide dissemination of new information. Paradoxically enough, though medical science is becoming more and more specialized, it is in some ways becoming more generalized as well. An embryologist today has much more in common with a biochemist than twenty years ago; so does a geneticist with a bacteriologist, and an immunologist with a physician. The "vertical" involvement in depth which any creative scientist must develop to make an original research contribution has gone hand in hand with a "horizontal" broadening of the base of each discipline, due to a general recognition of the interrelatedness of the biosciences. The emergence of planned interdisciplinary communications schemes, and their increasing effectiveness, has been one of the signal achievements of science in the last decade. Communication is a problem; there are gaps, but they are being tackled intelligently and successfully.

A final comment on hierarchies of scientific disciplines is warranted. There is a view, perhaps most forcefully expressed in the United States, that the only "fundamental" way of looking at biological phenomena is through the language of biochemistry. It is true that all bodily processes, and thus all human behavior and all manifestations of disease, rest on chemical events within cells and tissues. However, the vast bulk of observable events exhibited by mammalian species and studied through biological research are far too multifactorial and complex yet to be explicable in chemical terms. Thus there are hierarchical layers of understanding, each discipline resting on others more fundamental, but each possessing inherent validity and usefulness. Striving for the manifestly unattainable, scientists seek to create a steady continuum of knowledge. What really happens is a growth of scientific disciplines in two directions. Subjects like immunology, genetics, and cell biology grow internally; that is, new insights accumulate within the existing format of the discipline. They build bridges; that is, facts emerge which allow a principle of the discipline suddenly to be explained in the language of a more fundamental science, such as chemistry. Bridges extend "down" to chemistry and physics, but also "up" to behavioral science, clinical medicine, and demography. There is a certain danger in endowing biochemistry and molecular biology with a kind of *primus inter pares* status. The most efficient way for science to progress for both the practical benefit and intellectual enlightenment of mankind is along a broad front of related areas, moving ahead in close parallel formation.

What is the most welcome aspect of a career in science? The realization that the twin driving aims of satisfying man's thirst for knowledge and of improving his balance of power in the constant battle against his environment and the forces of nature can be achieved simultaneously. Every major advance in medical science contains these two elements, usually in equal measure. I do hope that this analysis of present-day immunology has provided some glimpse of the excitement and rich promise inherent in modern medical research. If so, my effort and yours have been worthwhile.

Suggestions for Further Reading

Reasonably Simple Books on Immunology and Related Subjects

Readings from Scientific American: *Immunology*. With introductions and additional material by F. M. Burnet. San Francisco: W. H. Freeman, 1976. *Scientific American* publishes popular science articles, of extremely high quality, usually contributed by a world leader in a particular field. The material is extensively edited to ensure readability and is very well illustrated. In this book, the key articles that have appeared on the subject of immunology in *Scientific American* have been brought together. The volume is of considerable historical interest, though of course some of the older articles now have a quaintly old-fashioned ring.

Burnet, F. M. *Self and Not-Self*. Melbourne: Melbourne University Press, and London: Cambridge University Press, 1969. This classic work summarizes cellular immunology as seen by one of its founding fathers.

Burnet, F. M., and D. O. White. *Natural History of Infectious Disease*. 4th ed. London: Cambridge University Press, 1972. This work traverses many of the problems at the interface of microbiology, immunology, and epidemiology.

Medawar, P. B. *The Uniqueness of the Individual*. London: Methuen, 1957. This is another classic work. It outlines the fundamental tenets of transplantation biology, with some interesting philosophical sidelights.

Cunningham, A. J. *Understanding Immunology*. New York and London: Academic Press, in press. This is a very recent book which attacks many of the problems of the present volume, but at a somewhat deeper level.

Fuller Textbooks

Roitt, I. *Essential Immunology*. 2d ed. Oxford: Blackwell Scientific Press, 1974. This is a textbook for medical students and covers the field briefly and well. The diagrams are particularly good. Inevitably for a book of only slightly more than 200 pages, there is a good deal of compression, but overall the book is very readable.

Humphrey, J. H. and R. G. White. *Immunology for Students of Medicine*. 3d ed. Oxford: Blackwell, 1970. This is a much longer textbook, used by many medical students and also by advanced science students; a high standard is maintained throughout. A fourth edition may be in the pipeline as this book goes to press.

Davis, B. D., et al. *Microbiology, Including Immunology and Molecular Genetics*. 2d ed. New York: Harper International, 1973. This American textbook is a wonderful compendium on a series of closely related fields in microbiology. Chapter 3 is on immunology, written in authoritative fashion by H. N. Eisen.

Review Publications

For those who wish to probe more deeply into specific aspects of immunology, particularly at the advancing edge of the field, a number of excellent review publications are available. The most widely read of these are *Advances in Immunology*, edited by F. J. Dixon and H. G. Kunkel, brought out annually by Academic Press, New York; and *Immunological Reviews* (formerly *Transplantation Reviews*) edited by G. Möller, published by Munksgaard, Copenhagen (several volumes of this publication come out each year).

The editors of *Advances in Immunology* also produce, at irregular intervals, an international series of monographs and treatises, published by Academic Press in New York and London. The first of these is by myself and G. L. Ada, *Antigens, Lymphoid Cells and the Immune Response* (1971). At least four other books in the series will be out by the time the present volume is printed.

INDEX